HAEMATOLOGY
A Core Curriculum

HAEMATOLOGY

A Core Curriculum

Barbara Jane Bain
Imperial College London, UK

Imperial College Press

Published by

Imperial College Press
57 Shelton Street
Covent Garden
London WC2H 9HE

Distributed by

World Scientific Publishing Co. Pte. Ltd.

5 Toh Tuck Link, Singapore 596224

USA office: 27 Warren Street, Suite 401-402, Hackensack, NJ 07601

UK office: 57 Shelton Street, Covent Garden, London WC2H 9HE

British Library Cataloguing-in-Publication Data
A catalogue record for this book is available from the British Library.

HAEMATOLOGY
A Core Curriculum
Copyright © 2010 by Imperial College Press

ISBN-13 978-1-84816-710-0
ISBN-10 1-84816-710-5
ISBN-13 978-1-84816-499-4 (pbk)
ISBN-10 1-84816-499-8 (pbk)

Typeset by Stallion Press
Email: enquiries@stallionpress.com

Printed by FulIsland Offset Printing (S) Pte Ltd. Singapore

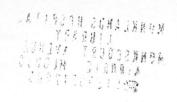

Contents

Preface

I should like to thank both colleagues from Imperial College and Imperial College Healthcare NHS Trust, who have kindly read the manuscript and made helpful suggestions, and other friends and colleagues, who have generously provided illustrations. Various chapters were critically reviewed by: Dr Saad Abdalla, Dr Ian Gabriel, Dr Ed Kanfer, Professor Mike Laffan, Professor David Lane, Dr Donald Macdonald, Dr Sasha Marks, Dr Carolyn Millar, Dr Jiří Pavlů, Dr Amin Rahemtulla, Dr Fiona Regan, Professor Irene Roberts, Dr Megan Rowley, Dr Nina Salooja and Dr Abdul Shlebak.

Illustrations were kindly provided by: Dr Abbas Hashim Abdulsalam, Al-yarmouk Teaching Hospital, Baghdad; Dr Saad Abdalla, St Mary's Hospital, London; Emeritus Professor Daniel Catovsky, Royal Marsden Hospital, London; Professor Mike Laffan, Hammersmith Hospital, London; Dr Julie McCarthy, Cork University Hospital; Dr Alistair Reid, Hammersmith Hospital, London; Dr Helen Wordsworth, Sullivan Nicolaides Pathology, Brisbane; Marketing Department, NHS Blood and Transplant; Professor Geoffrey Pasvol, Imperial College, London; Dr Andrew Wotherspoon, Royal Marsden Hospital, London; and Dr Christine Wright, City Hospital, Birmingham.

1

Physiology of the Blood and Bone Marrow

What Do You Have to Know?

☞ Which cells are normally present in the blood and what is their function
☞ The normal intravascular life span of erythrocytes, neutrophils and platelets
☞ Where and how blood cells are produced
☞ The production and function of erythropoietin
☞ The source and absorption of iron, vitamin B_{12} and folic acid, and their role in haemopoiesis

Blood Cells and Their Functions

The circulating blood contains red cells, white cells and platelets suspended in plasma (Fig. 1.1). The cells in the circulating blood originate in the bone marrow.

Red cells, also known as **erythrocytes**, differ from most body cells in that they no longer have a nucleus. This is extruded when they leave the bone marrow. Normal mature red cells are disc-shaped and, because they lack a nucleus, are flexible; they can deform and squeeze though capillaries. The major function of the red cell is the transport of oxygen from the

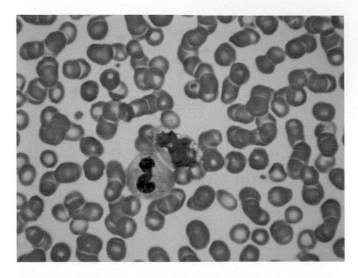

Fig. 1.1. A stained blood film showing erythrocytes, leucocytes (a neutrophil and a monocyte) and platelets.

lungs to peripheral tissues but it also transports CO_2 from the tissues to the lungs and has a role in nitric oxide (NO) transport and metabolism, favouring generation of NO and vasodilation in conditions of hypoxia.

The principal constituent of the red cell, responsible for oxygen transport and contributing to CO_2 transport and interactions with NO, is haemoglobin. It is an iron-containing protein composed of four polypeptide chains known as globin chains, each of which has a deep pocket into which an iron-containing haem group is inserted. The tetrameric haemoglobin molecule is composed of two heterodimers: in normal adult haemoglobin (haemoglobin A) the dimer is composed of an α and a β chain (Fig. 1.2). Oxygen for transport can enter the haem pocket and bind reversibly to haem. The globin chains can alter their relationship to each other in response to uptake or release of oxygen by haem. The loss of the oxygen molecule from one haem makes it more likely that other oxygen molecules will be lost from other haems. This is known as co-operativity and is responsible for the sigmoid shape of the oxygen dissociation curve (Fig. 1.3). Co-operativity ensures that haemoglobin takes up oxygen readily as it passes through the lungs, becoming almost fully saturated but, when it reaches tissues, oxygen is equally readily released. Delivery of

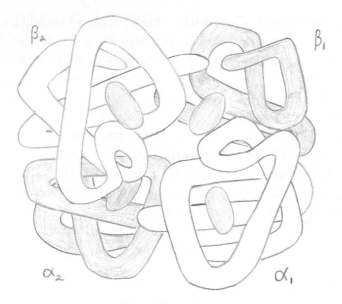

Fig. 1.2. A diagram of a haemoglobin molecule, showing two α and two β globin chains, each with a haem in the haem pocket. The $\alpha_1\beta_1$ dimer is shown in pink and the $\alpha_2\beta_2$ dimer in blue. The haem group is represented in green.

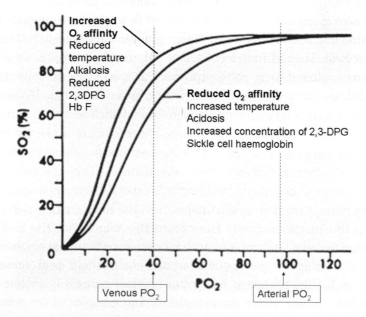

Fig. 1.3. The oxygen dissociation curve illustrating the sigmoid curve that results from co-operativity.

oxygen in the tissues is facilitated by a higher temperature and a lower pH so that more oxygen is available to metabolically-active tissues. It is also facilitated by interaction with 2,3 diphosphoglycerate (2,3 DPG), a glycolytic intermediate that increases in concentration in response to anaemia. Higher temperature, lower pH and a higher concentration of 2,3 DPG thus decrease the affinity of haemoglobin for oxygen.

Erythrocytes are enclosed by a surface membrane, which is a lipid bilayer, supported by a cytoskeleton that maintains the biconcave shape of the cell. They contain enzymes of the Emden-Meyerhoff (or glycolytic) pathway, which meets the energy needs of the cell and enzymes of the pentose (hexosemonophosphate) shunt, which protects the cell from oxidant damage. The erythrocyte life span is about 120 days, effete cells being removed by macrophages, particularly in the spleen. The synthesis of haemoglobin is discussed further in Chapter 5 and the red cell membrane and enzymes in Chapter 6.

White cells, also known as **leucocytes**, defend the body against infection and participate in immune responses. Those that are normally present in the blood are of five types. Three of these are referred to as **granulocytes**, because their cytoplasm contains granules; depending on the colour of the granules in a stained blood film they can be divided into neutrophils (small lilac granules), eosinophils (larger orange granules) and basophils (large purple granules). They all have lobulated or polymorphous nuclei and thus are sometimes referred to as polymorphonuclear leucocytes or 'polymorphs.' Granulocytes function mainly in the tissues, rather than in the bloodstream. They reach tissues by migrating through the endothelium of capillaries.

Neutrophils (Fig. 1.4a) spend only about 7 hours in the circulation. They are phagocytic cells that respond to chemotactic stimuli by migrating to sites of infection, inflammation or cell death. This process involves rolling along the endothelium, adhering to specific endothelial receptors, moving through capillary walls (diapedesis) and migrating through tissues in response to chemotaxins. The neutrophils engulf bacteria and other unwanted material within tissues by a process known as phagocytosis. This involves flowing of pseudopodia around the particle with subsequent fusion so that the unwanted bacterium or other particle is enclosed in a phagocytic vacuole within the cytoplasm. The granules of the neutrophil (which contain proteolytic enzymes and myeloperoxidase) are then

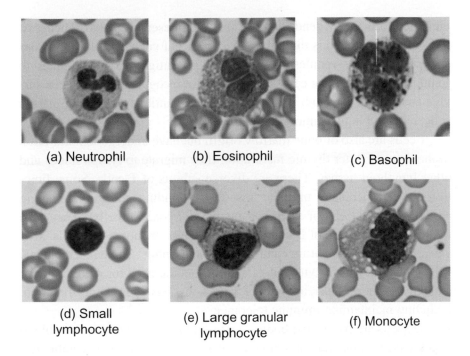

(a) Neutrophil   (b) Eosinophil   (c) Basophil

(d) Small lymphocyte   (e) Large granular lymphocyte   (f) Monocyte

Fig. 1.4. Normal leucocytes in the peripheral blood: (a) a neutrophil; (b) an eosinophil; (c) a basophil; (d) a small lymphocyte; (e) a large granular lymphocyte; (f) a monocyte.

discharged into the phagocytic vacuole, where H_2O_2 and other reactive oxygen species are generated. The result is killing of microbes and proteolysis of phagosome contents. Neutrophils spend about 30 hours in tissues.

The major function of **eosinophils** (Fig. 1.4b) is defence against parasitic infection. They are less efficient than neutrophils in defence against bacteria. In addition to these beneficial functions, eosinophils have unwanted actions when they are involved in allergic reactions. **Basophils** (Fig. 1.4c) also participate in defence against parasites and allergic responses.

Lymphocytes (Figs. 1.4d, e) are smaller than granulocytes and have a round nucleus. A minority of them have a small number of cytoplasmic granules. Circulating lymphocytes look very similar to each other but include cells of three lineages, B cells, T cells and natural killer (NK) cells. B cells are of bone marrow origin. They migrate from the bloodstream to lymph nodes or other lymphoid tissues where they are exposed to antigens

presented to them by dendritic cells (antigen-presenting cells). Their exit
from the bloodstream is through high endothelial venules of lymph nodes
and post-capillary venules of other tissues. Antigen exposure leads to
somatic mutation so that cells most capable of recognising the antigen survive and mature into both memory B cells and antibody-secreting plasma
cells, responsible for humoral immunity.

T cells are also of bone marrow origin but have undergone maturation
in the thymus. After thymic maturation they migrate to lymph nodes and
other lymphoid tissues. There are diverse subsets of T cells. Some function in cell-mediated immune responses, binding to and damaging
antibody-coated cells or microorganisms (cytotoxic T cells). They also
modulate the function of B cells, acting as helper or suppressor cells, activate macrophages and attract and activate neutrophils. Some resemble NK
cells in that they have cytotoxic effect without the need for recognition of
an antigen. There is also a subset of T cells that has a regulatory function,
including maintaining immune tolerance.

NK cells are part of the body's innate immune response, being able to
attack cancer cells and foreign cells even though they are not antibody-
coated. Lymphocytes that contain granules are either NK cells or cytotoxic
T cells. Otherwise it is not possible to distinguish T cells from B cells by
their appearance in the blood film. Lymphocytes recirculate between the
lymphatic system and the bloodstream. They spend a very variable period
of time in the circulation. Their survival is very variable but in some cases
this may amount to many years.

Monocytes (Fig. 1.4f) are the largest cells normally present in the blood.
They have a lobulated nucleus and plentiful cytoplasm. They spend several
days in the circulation but their main function is in the tissues. There they
mature into macrophages or histiocytes (collectively known as the reticu-
loendothelial system), capable of phagocytosing and killing microorganisms
and breaking down and removing cellular debris. They present antigens to
lymphocytes. Whereas neutrophils are most important in defence against
acute bacterial infection, cells of the monocyte/macrophage lineage are most
important in defence against chronic bacterial infections, such as tuberculosis, and in chronic fungal infections. They also secrete numerous cytokines
that enhance the inflammatory response to infection and also growth factors
that promote the production of neutrophils and monocytes. In addition,

macrophages remove parasites (such as malaria parasites) and other particles from red cells. They destroy red cells at the end of their life span and store the iron released from haemoglobin so that it can be recycled.

Platelets are small particles formed by fragmentation of the cytoplasm of bone marrow megakaryocytes. They function in the primary haemostatic response, forming a platelet plug at the site of small vessel injury. When activated, they also expose altered phospholipid on their surfaces that interacts with coagulation factors to promote blood coagulation at the site of tissue injury. They survive for about 10 days in the circulation.

Bone Marrow Cells and Normal Haemopoiesis

All the blood cells are ultimately derived, in the bone marrow, from a pluripotent haemopoietic stem cell that is capable of giving rise to both lymphoid and myeloid progeny via a common lymphoid progenitor cell and a common myeloid progenitor cell respectively (Fig. 1.5). The common lymphoid progenitor gives rise to B cells, T cells and NK cells. The common

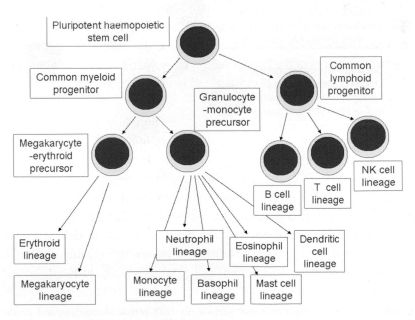

Fig. 1.5. The haemopoietic stem cell hierarchy.

myeloid progenitor is a multipotent haemopoietic progenitor cell (sometimes also known as a multipotent myeloid stem cell) capable of giving rise to cells of all myeloid lineages. It gives rise initially to an erythroid-megakaryocyte progenitor cell and to a granulocyte-monocyte progenitor cell. The granulocyte-monocyte progenitor gives rise not only to monocytes and the three types of granulocyte, but also to the antigen-presenting dendritic cells and to mast cells, which are tissue cells concerned with immune responses. The monocyte/macrophage lineage gives rise to many specialised tissue macrophages (e.g. Kupffer cells in the liver) and also to osteoclasts, giant cells needed for the breakdown and remodelling of bone.

Haemopoietic stem cells have as a defining quality the ability to reproduce themselves and also to differentiate into progenitor cells of specific lineages that ultimately give rise to mature end cells (Fig. 1.6). Progenitor cells and their progeny undergo a series of cell divisions associated with maturation (Fig. 1.7). In the case of the megakaryocyte lineage, there is

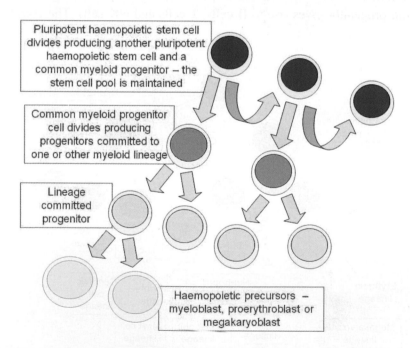

Pluripotent haemopoietic stem cell divides producing another pluripotent haemopoietic stem cell and a common myeloid progenitor – the stem cell pool is maintained

Common myeloid progenitor cell divides producing progenitors committed to one or other myeloid lineage

Lineage committed progenitor

Haemopoietic precursors – myeloblast, proerythroblast or megakaryoblast

Fig. 1.6.   A diagram illustrating that stem cells both renew themselves and produce differentiated progeny.

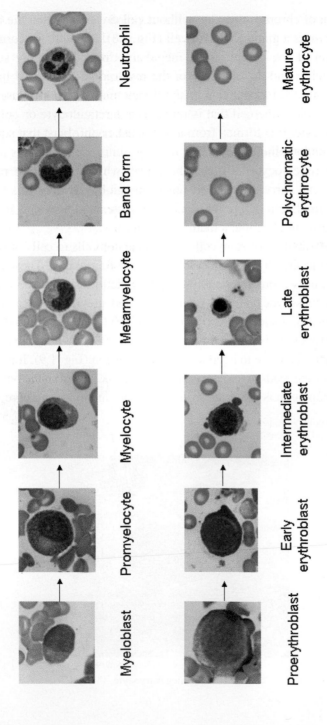

Fig. 1.7. The stages of maturation of erythroid and granulocyte progenitors to mature cells.

reduplication of chromosomes but without cell division so that the mature megakaryocyte is a giant polyploid cell (Fig. 1.8). Platelets are formed by fragmentation of the cytoplasm of megakaryocytes. In healthy subjects only the platelets and the end cells of the myeloid and erythroid lineages are released into the bloodstream in significant numbers. In the case of the erythrocyte lineage, the cell that is released is a reticulocyte or polychromatic erythrocyte. It is formed from a nucleated erythroblast that squeezes through the endothelium into a bone marrow sinusoid, leaving its nucleus behind. The reticulocyte still has ribosomes (which the mature red cell does not) so can carry on synthesising haemoglobin. It does this for 1–3 days in the circulation before it loses its ribosomes and remodels its shape to that of a disc and become a mature red cell.

The differentiation of stem cells and progenitor cells to cells of specific lineages is controlled by a considerable number of cytokines. These include stem cell factor, various interleukins, erythropoietin (erythrocytes), thrombopoietin (megakaryocytes) and granulocyte and granulocyte-macrophage colony-stimulating factors (G-CSF and GM-CSF) (granulocytes and monocytes). Erythropoietin is produced mainly (about 90%) by juxtatubular cells in the kidney in response to a reduced oxygen tension (Fig. 1.9). It increases erythropoiesis and leads to earlier release of reticulocytes from the bone marrow. Thrombopoietin is produced by the liver (production being upregulated

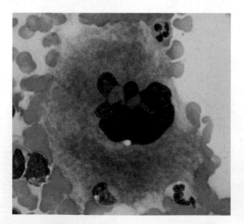

Fig. 1.8. A megakaryocyte.

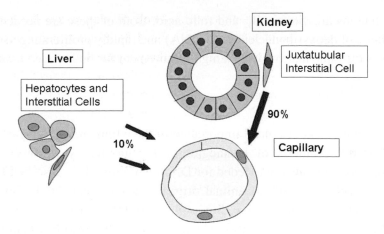

Fig. 1.9. Diagram showing production of erythropoietin by renal and, to a lesser extent, hepatic cells.

by infection, inflammation and iron deficiency) and in small amounts by bone marrow stromal cells (production being upregulated by severe thrombocytopenia). Thrombopoietin combines with a specific receptor on cell membranes. It enhances survival and expansion of haemopoietic stem cells and promotes differentiation of these cells to megakaryocytes. G-CSF is produced by fibroblasts, endothelial cells and macrophages; it increases neutrophil production, survival and functional activity, and accelerates release of neutrophils from the bone marrow. GM-CSF is produced by lymphocytes and macrophages; it increases the proliferation of progenitor cells, accelerates production and release from the bone marrow of neutrophils and monocytes, and increases the functional activity of both cell types.

In the adult, the haemopoietic marrow (red marrow) is found mainly in the skull, sternum, ribs, vertebrae, upper sacrum, pelvis and proximal long bones. Marrow that is haemopoietically inactive is composed largely of fat (yellow marrow). In children the red marrow extends through a much larger proportion of the skeleton, e.g. into the distal long bones. In adults, under conditions of sustained need for more blood cells (particularly red cells), the red marrow can re-expand into more distal parts of the skeleton.

Normal haemopoiesis requires a supply of amino acids and also various vitamins and minerals. The most important of the minerals is iron, which is an essential constituent of haemoglobin. The most important of the vitamins are vitamin B_{12} and folic acid. Both of these are needed for synthesis of deoxyribonucleic acid (DNA) and rapidly proliferating tissues such as the bone marrow have a high requirement for both these vitamins.

Iron

Iron is an element of crucial importance in the human body, being essential for the synthesis of haemoglobin, myoglobin, cytochromes and ribonucleotide reductase (needed for DNA synthesis). It is absorbed from the diet with foodstuffs of animal origin (e.g. red meat, offal, fish and eggs) being the richest source. Some plant products, such as lentils, also contain a useful amount of iron. Haem iron is better absorbed than non-haem iron (about 10% can be absorbed in contrast with only 1–2%). Very little iron is normally lost from the body. What is lost is in desquamating cells from the skin or gastrointestinal tract or in the red cells of blood. Uptake of about 1 mg a day is needed in adult men while menstruating women need about 2 mg a day. Pregnant women have a high requirement and lactation also increases need. Growing infants, children and adolescents have a greater requirement than adult men. Premature babies have increased iron needs as around half of the transfer of iron from the mother to the fetus is in the last month of intrauterine life. Blood donation increases the need for iron by 0.7 mg/day for each unit donated in a year so that men and women donating three times a year would have a daily requirement of 3 and 4 mg respectively. Since normally only about 10% of dietary iron is absorbed, the dietary iron intake needs to be considerably higher than the body's needs.

Iron is released from food in the stomach through the action of peptic enzymes and gastric acid. Iron passes into the duodenum where absorption is maximal. Some absorption also occurs in the jejunum. Any ferric (Fe^{+++}) iron is first converted to the ferrous form (Fe^{++}) by a membrane enzyme, duodenal cytochrome B (Fig. 1.10). Ferrous iron is then able to bind to the membrane divalent metal transporter 1 to enter the enterocyte. To be absorbed into the body, iron must pass right through the enterocyte, exiting by means of membrane ferroportin, so that it can be delivered to plasma transferrin. This requires reconversion to the ferric form, achieved with the help of several other co-operating proteins. If export from the cell

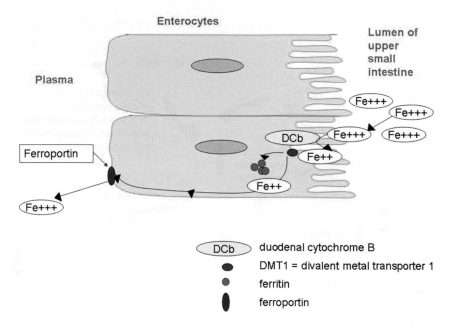

Fig. 1.10. The absorption of iron by mucosal cells of the upper intestine, particularly the duodenum.

does not occur, iron is converted to ferritin and is lost to the body when the enterocyte is shed into the gut lumen.

Since the body has no effective means of getting rid of excess iron, the rate of absorption must be carefully controlled. This is achieved by means of hepcidin, a protein synthesised by the liver. When body stores of iron are low, hepcidin synthesis is low and iron absorption is facilitated. In conditions of iron excess, hepcidin is synthesised in increased amounts and this leads to ferroportin of enterocytes being internalised and degraded (Fig. 1.11). Iron then cannot pass through the cell so is lost to the body when the cells are shed. When there is iron deficiency, much less hepcidin is synthesised and iron absorption is promoted.

Hepcidin has another role in maintaining plasma iron for delivery to erythroid precursors and other cells. The iron stored in macrophages in the form of haemosiderin can be mobilised and, by means of ferroportin, exported from the cell to the plasma. In the macrophage, as in the enterocyte, hepcidin leads to internalisation and degradation of ferroportin so that

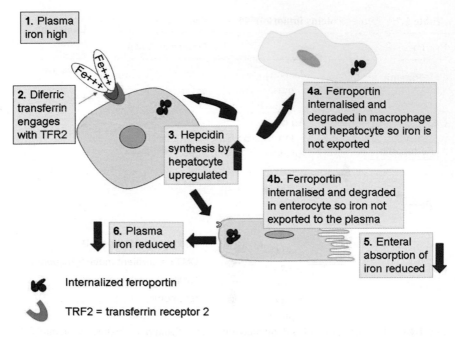

Fig. 1.11. The control of iron absorption and release from stores by hepcidin when plasma iron is high.

iron is trapped in the macrophage. In summary, in iron deficiency or depletion, when little hepcidin is synthesised, both macrophage export and intestinal absorption of iron are promoted. This maximises the iron available for erythropoiesis. Conversely, if iron is replete and more hepcidin is synthesised, iron stays in macrophages and is not absorbed by the intestine.

The iron that is conserved in the body is in the form of haemosiderin within macrophages, referred to as the iron stores. Body iron can be viewed as belonging to three pools: the functional pool, such as haemoglobin and myoglobin (about 2–3 g); the storage pool of ferritin and haemosiderin (about 1 g); and the transit pool of iron bound to transferrin in the plasma (only about 3 mg but functionally very important).

The difference between iron deficiency and iron depletion is that in deficiency the amount of iron available to tissues is inadequate for haemoglobin synthesis whereas in depletion the iron stores are reduced or absent but absorption is keeping up with the body's needs. The roles of

Table 1.1. Some proteins important in iron absorption, transport and utilisation.

Protein	Nature and role
Duodenal cytochrome b	An enterocyte luminal membrane protein that converts ferric iron (Fe^{+++}) to ferrous (Fe^{++}) so that it can be absorbed
Divalent metal transporter 1	An enterocyte luminal membrane protein that transports ferrous iron into the enterocyte
Ferroportin	An enterocyte basal membrane protein and macrophage membrane protein that transports iron out of enterocytes and macrophages to the plasma
Transferrin	A plasma protein that accepts iron from ferroportin of enterocytes or macrophages and delivers it to erythroid precursors and other cells; it binds to transferrin receptors on the cell membrane and the iron transferrin complex is then internalised with the transferrin and its receptor subsequently being recycled to the cell surface
Hepcidin	A peptide hormone synthesised by the liver that controls plasma iron by reducing iron absorption and promoting retention of iron in macrophages when iron is plentiful
Ferritin	A cytoplasmic protein, a storage form of iron, present in many cells
Haemosiderin	A cytoplasmic protein, a storage form of iron, formed from ferritin and mainly present in macrophages

some proteins important in iron transport and storage are summarised in Table 1.1.

Vitamin B_{12}

Vitamin B_{12} is derived from animal products in the diet. A vegetarian diet therefore has a reduced B_{12} content whereas a vegan diet has negligible B_{12} and requires supplementation. The daily requirement is about 1 μg and, since not all is absorbed, an intake of 2.4 μg is advised. The main loss of B_{12} from the body is in the bile where only about half of the 1.4 μg secreted each day is resorbed — and less if there is a defect in absorption. Dietary vitamin B_{12} is released from food by the action of hydrochloric acid and peptic enzymes. It binds to intrinsic factor (secreted by the stomach) in the duodenum and the B_{12}-intrinsic factor complex is then internalised by ileal cells. The process is quite complex and is illustrated in Figs. 1.12 and 1.13. In the plasma, B_{12} is transported and delivered to the cells by transcobalamin. It is also bound to haptocorrin, of uncertain function, but this protein is not capable of delivering it to cells.

Vitamin B_{12} is essential for two metabolic pathways. It is a coenzyme in the conversion of 5-methyl-tetrahydrofolate to tetrahydrofolate and the simultaneous conversion of homocysteine to methionine; this pathway is essential for synthesis of DNA and RNA. It is also a coenzyme for the synthesis of succinyl coenzyme A, a necessary step in catabolism of some fatty acids and some amino acids. Because of its role in DNA synthesis the effects of any deficiency of vitamin B_{12} are prominent in rapidly-dividing tissues, such as the bone marrow.

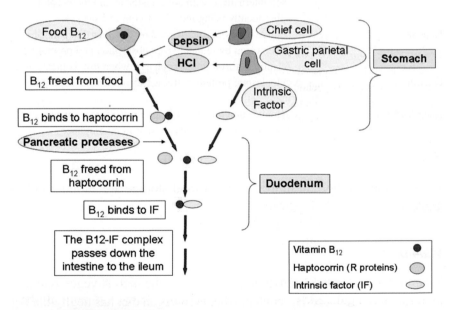

Fig. 1.12. The gastric and duodenal stages of vitamin B_{12} absorption: food containing vitamin B_{12} is digested in the stomach by means of hydrochloric acid and pepsin secreted by gastric cells; B_{12} is freed and combines with haptocorrin (of salivary gland origin); the B_{12}-haptocorrin complex passes into the duodenum where the action of pancreatic proteases and the higher pH lead to the B_{12} being released from haptocorrin and combining with intrinsic factor, also of gastric origin; the B_{12}-intrinsic factor complex passes down the intestine to the ileum where absorption occurs.

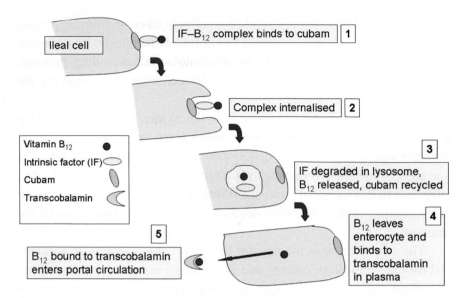

Fig. 1.13. The ileal stage of vitamin B_{12} absorption: the intrinsic factor (IF)-B_{12} complex binds to cubam, an IF receptor on the surface membrane of ileal cells; the IF-B_{12} complex is internalised; the complex dissociates with IF being degraded, cubam being recycled to the cell surface and B_{12} being exported form the cell to the plasma where it is bound to transcobalamin; transcobalamin delivers B_{12} to hepatocytes for storage and to body cells that require it for DNA synthesis.

Folic acid

Folic acid is derived from the diet. Rich dietary sources include fruit and vegetables (particularly green vegetables), liver, kidney, yeast and yeast extracts. In some countries (e.g. the USA and Canada) flour is fortified with folic acid. Folic acid refers specifically to pteroylglutamic acid (a monoglutamate form) but most dietary folate is in the form of polyglutamates. The folate within body cells is also mainly in the form of polyglutamates with three to seven glutamic acid residues. The term 'folate' refers to all these forms of folic acid.

Dietary folate is absorbed maximally in the upper jejunum. Polyglutamates must first be deconjugated to folic acid. This happens at the brush border but whether in the lumen or within the cell is not clear. Absorption is an active process. Folic acid that is absorbed into the enterocyte is mainly converted to methyl-tetrahydrofolate before being exported to the plasma. Methyl-tetrahydrofolate is actively taken up from the plasma by cells. Within cells it is converted to a polyglutamate form. This conversion, plus the binding of folate to intracellular folate-binding proteins, means that the folate is retained within the cell where it is required for various metabolic processes.

The daily requirement of folate is about 50 μg. About half of dietary folate is absorbed. The minimum recommended daily intake is 400 μg with the average diet containing 400–600 μg. Folate is stored in the liver and can be mobilised from there to other tissues. Body stores are 5–10 mg, sufficient to last for about 4 months if intake stops. Folate is lost from the body in urine, in the bile and in desquamating cells from the skin and the intestine.

The role of folate is the transfer of single carbon groups. It is essential for the synthesis of purines and pyrimidines and for interconversions of various amino acids. The body can compensate for reduced purine synthesis by reducing the rate of degradation but if pyrimidine synthesis is reduced there is a reduced rate of synthesis of DNA with serious pathological effects, affecting particularly haemopoietic cells and other rapidly dividing cells.

The mechanism of megaloblastic anaemia in vitamin B_{12} deficiency is actually a functional folate deficiency. When B_{12} is deficient there is reduced conversion of 5-methyl-tetrathydrofolate to tetrahydrofolate, the form that can be polyglutamated and can participate in pathways leading to DNA and RNA synthesis. Providing extra folic acid can correct this defect in B_{12}-deficient patients but without there being any effect of the independent adenosylcobalamin pathway, which is involved in the methylation of myelin. The haematological but not the neurological effects of vitamin B_{12} deficiency can thus be improved by folic acid.

Other essential requirements for haemopoiesis

Normal haemopoiesis requires a supply of amino acids and energy so that protein-energy malnutrition leads to anaemia. Various growth factors are also essential but in general these are not rate-limiting. However erythropoietin is of critical importance for erythropoiesis and reduced synthesis in renal failure leads to anaemia. There is also a requirement for normal levels of hormones such as growth hormone, thyroxine, adrenal steroids and androgens so that anaemia is a feature of hypopituitarism, hypothyroidism, Addison's disease and hypogonadism in men. In addition there is a requirement for copper, vitamin C, vitamin B_6 (pyridoxine) and vitamin B_2 (riboflavin). However, deficiency of any of these haematinics is quite uncommon as a cause of anaemia or other cytopenia.

Conclusions

Production and destruction of blood cells is finely balanced and is maintained throughout life. Production is controlled by growth factors and cytokines and can be increased in response to increased needs. Normal haemopoiesis requires normal numbers of haemopoietic stem cells in an appropriate microenvironment, normal concentrations of various hormones and availability of amino acids, iron and various vitamins. The major functions of blood cells are oxygen transport and defence against infection.

2

The Blood Count and Film

What Do You Have to Know?

☞ The constituent parts of a blood count

☞ The meaning and clinical significance of a reticulocyte count

☞ The meaning of the words that are frequently used to describe abnormalities in the blood count and blood film and their possible clinical significance

☞ The meaning of 'normal range' and 'reference range'

☞ The approximate normal ranges for the white cell count, haemoglobin concentration, mean cell volume and platelet count in healthy adults

☞ How to interpret a blood count and develop a differential diagnosis

☞ The meaning and clinical significance of an 'erythrocyte sedimentation rate'

The Full Blood Count

The term 'full blood count' (FBC) refers to a group of tests performed simultaneously on a blood sample to assess whether there is any haematological abnormality. The tests that are almost always included in an FBC are shown in Table 2.1. In modern haematological practice these tests are performed on large automated analysers capable of processing many hundreds of samples in a day. Further tests are sometimes also included. The

Table 2.1.   The full blood count.

Test	Abbreviation	Units	Normal range in men*	Normal range in women*
White blood cell count	WBC	$\times 10^9$/l	3.7–9.5	3.9–11.1
Red blood cell count	RBC	$\times 10^{12}$/l	4.32–5.66	3.88–4.99
Haemoglobin concentration	Hb	g/dl	13.3–16.7	11.8–14.8
Haematocrit	Hct	l/l	0.39–0.50	0.36–0.44
Mean cell volume	MCV	fl	82–98	
Mean cell haemoglobin	MCH	pg	27.3–32.6	
Mean cell haemoglobin concentration	MCHC	g/dl	31.6–34.9	
Platelet count		$\times 10^9$/l	168–411[†]	188–445[†]

* From Bain, B.J. (2006). *Blood Cells*. Fourth Edition. Blackwell Publishing, Oxford.
[†] Reported ranges from different instruments vary.

blood count is performed on a blood specimen that has been anticoagulated by being mixed with ethylene diaminetetra-acetic acid (EDTA), a chelating agent that prevents clotting by binding calcium. If you are obtaining a blood specimen from a patient for an FBC be sure to use a tube containing EDTA, add the correct volume of blood and mix the blood sample with the anticoagulant.

The white blood cell count

The white blood cell count (WBC, also known as the white cell count) was initially determined by counting cells using a microscope and a glass counting chamber. Nowadays it is counted by an automated instrument that detects individual cells flowing in a stream through a sensor. Recognition is either because the cell interrupts a beam of light or because it alters the electrical current flowing between two electrodes. A WBC is performed on a sample in which the mature red cells have been lysed by solutions to which they are exposed within the instrument so that the only cells that will be counted are the white cells and any nucleated red blood cells that might be present.

The red blood cell count

The red blood cell count (RBC, also known as the red cell count) was initially determined with a counting chamber. As for the WBC, it is now determined by an instrument that counts red cells flowing through a sensor. However, this time the red cells are not lysed. White cells will actually also be included in the count but because they are infrequent in relation to the red cells this does not usually introduce much error.

The haemoglobin concentration

The haemoglobin concentration (Hb) is determined by lysing red cells and measuring light transmitted through a diluted sample of the blood at a specific wavelength after conversion of the haemoglobin to a stable form.

The haematocrit

It is possible to measure the proportion of red cells in an anticoagulated blood sample by centrifuging a tube of the blood and comparing the height of the column of red cells with the total height of the blood sample. This test is called a packed cell volume (PCV). It is no longer performed because it is not suitable for dealing with large numbers of blood specimens. The modern equivalent is called a haematocrit (Hct). It has the same significance as a PCV but instruments calculate it rather than measuring it directly. This is done by multiplying the average size of a red cell, the mean cell volume (MCV), by the number of red cells in a litre of blood (the RBC).

The mean cell volume

The mean cell volume (MCV) was once estimated by dividing the PCV (obtained by centrifugation) by the RBC (from a counting chamber). This was a very laborious technique so it was not done very often. Modern instruments estimate the MCV from the height of the electrical impulse generated by interruption of a light beam or an electrical current. The same electrical impulse is therefore used both to count the cells and to size them.

The mean cell haemoglobin

The mean cell haemoglobin (MCH) is the average **amount** of haemoglobin in an individual red cell. Instruments calculate it by dividing the haemoglobin in a given volume of blood by the number of red cells in the same volume.

The mean cell haemoglobin concentration

The mean cell haemoglobin concentration (MCHC) is the average **concentration** of haemoglobin, rather than the absolute amount, in an individual red cell. Fig. 2.1 is a visual representation of the difference between the MCH and the MCHC. Instruments calculate it by dividing the haemoglobin in a given volume of blood by the proportion of the whole blood sample that is occupied by red cells.

The red cell distribution width

The red cell distribution width (RDW) is a measurement of the amount of variation in the size of the red cells.

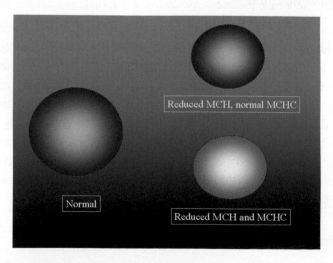

Fig. 2.1. A diagram to illustrate the difference between the mean cell haemoglobin (MCH) and the mean cell haemoglobin concentration (MCHC).

The platelet count

Platelets are counted by the same principles as red cells and white cells. They can be distinguished from red and white cells by their smaller size.

The red cell indices

The term 'red cells indices' refers to the RBC, MCV, MCH and MCHC. The formulae (which you do not need to know) for calculating the latter three values are:

$$MCV \text{ (fl)} = \frac{PCV \text{ (l/l)} \times 1000}{RBC \text{ (cells/l)} \times 10^{-12}}$$

$$MCH \text{ (pg)} = \frac{Hb \text{ (g/dl)} \times 10}{RBC \text{ (cells/l)} \times 10^{-12}}$$

$$MCHC \text{ (g/dl)} = \frac{Hb \text{ (g/dl)}}{PCV \text{ (l/l)}}$$

The red cell indices are very useful for indicating the likely cause of anaemia.

The reticulocyte count

A reticulocyte count is a supplement to an FBC, rather than a normal part of it. It can be performed using a microscope, counting the percentage of erythrocytes that have developed a 'reticulum' or network of precipitated dye after incubation of the blood sample with a dye such as methylene blue (Fig. 2.2). This is a method for identifying ribonucleic acid (RNA) within red cells, thus demonstrating that these are cells newly released from the bone marrow (1–3 days old). Reticulocyte counts can also be performed by automated instruments, using either the same principle as the reticulocyte count with a microscope or alternatively, using a fluorescent dye that binds to RNA.

The Differential White Cell Count

The different types of white cell can be distinguished from each other by examining a stained blood film. If a hundred cells are counted and the

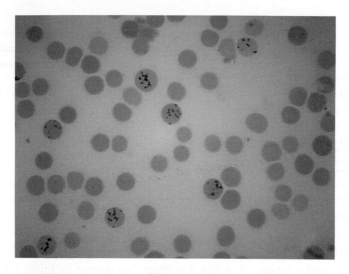

Fig. 2.2. A reticulocyte preparation, showing a reticulum of precipitated dye following incubation of blood with methylene blue.

percentages are multiplied by the WBC, the absolute number of cells of each type can be calculated. Calculating the percentage or absolute number of each cell type is referred to as a differential count. It is much more useful to calculate the absolute count than to try to make deductions from the percentages. For example, if a patient had 5% neutrophils and 95% lymphocytes this could indicate either a severe reduction of neutrophils or a marked increase in lymphocytes.

Many automated instruments can recognise the five normal types of white cell and can detect the presence of nucleated red blood cells (NRBC) and other cells that are not normally present in the circulating blood. If only normal cells are present they are capable of performing a differential count. If abnormal cells are present it is usually still necessary to perform a differential count on a blood film. However, some instruments are also capable of counting NRBC. Normal ranges for the differential white cell count are shown in Table 2.2.

Haematological Terminology

Haematologists use precise terms to refer to abnormalities in the blood count and film. Since they use these terms to report abnormalities to

Table 2.2.   The differential white cell count.

Test	Units	Normal range in men*	Normal range in women*
Neutrophil count	$\times 10^9$/l	1.7–6.1	1.7–7.5
Lymphocyte count	$\times 10^9$/l	1.0–3.2	
Monocyte count	$\times 10^9$/l	0.2–0.6	
Eosinophil count	$\times 10^9$/l	0.03–0.46	
Basophil count	$\times 10^9$/l	0.09–0.29	

*From Bain, B.J. (2006). *Blood Cells*. Fourth Edition. Blackwell Publishing, Oxford. Figures are for an automated instrument and will differ slightly between instruments; figures for manual differential counts will have broader limits.

clinical staff it is necessary for all doctors to understand them. The terms used to describe quantitative abnormalities are shown in Table 2.3; unfortunately these terms are not necessarily logical or consistent so you just have to learn how they are used. The terms used to describe erythrocytes and their abnormalities are shown and illustrated in Table 2.4.

Normal Ranges and Reference Ranges

Once we have got a laboratory result how do we know if it is normal? Laboratories issue test results with a reference range or normal range for comparison. A reference range is derived from a carefully defined population, the reference population: the definition will include the age and gender of the subjects and sometimes the ethnic origin or other relevant details. If a requirement to be in good health is part of the definition then a 'reference range' becomes a 'normal range'. Conventionally, reference ranges and normal ranges include the central 95% of results from the reference population. Ideally, tests would give a clear separation of healthy subjects (the normal range) and an unhealthy population, as shown in Fig. 2.3a. More often, the situation will be as shown in Fig. 2.3c, with a small amount of overlap between sick and well people. Sometimes a test gives poor separation of sick and well (Fig. 2.3b). Either the laboratory or the clinician looking after the patient has to decide the threshold to accept. If the figure chosen includes all sick people then a lot of normal people will also be included; the test becomes sensitive but at the cost of a high rate of false positives. If the threshold is moved down so that no healthy person is

Table 2.3. Terminology used for describing quantitative abnormalities in blood counts.

Term	Meaning
Anaemia	Reduced Hb
Polycythaemia or erythrocytosis	Either term can be used to indicate an increase in the RBC, Hb and Hct
Leucocytosis	Increased WBC
Leucopenia	Reduced WBC
Thrombocytosis	Increased platelet count
Thrombocytopenia	Reduced platelet count
Neutrophilia	Increased neutrophil count
Neutropenia	Reduced neutrophil count
Lymphocytosis	Increased lymphocyte count
Lymphopenia* or lymphocytopenia	Reduced lymphocyte count
Monocytosis	Increased monocyte count
Eosinophilia	Increased eosinophil count
Basophilia[†]	Increased basophil count
Reticulocytosis	Increased reticulocyte count
Reticulocytopenia	Reduced reticulocyte count

*The term 'lymphopenia' is particularly illogical because it is used to mean a reduced lymphocyte count not a reduced amount of lymph.

[†] Basophilia has a quite different alternative meaning; it also means an increased uptake of basic dyes by the cytoplasm of a cell so that when examined with a microscope it appears blue.

Table 2.4. Terminology used for describing erythrocytes and their abnormalities.

Term	Significance	Picture
Normocytic Normochromic	Of normal size With normal staining characteristics	
Anisocytosis	Increased variation in size	
Poikilocyte Poikilocytosis	An erythrocyte of abnormal shape Increased variation in shape	
Microcyte Microcytosis	Smaller than normal The presence of microcytes	

(Continued)

Table 2.4. *(Continued)*

Term	Significance	Picture
Macrocyte Macrocytosis	Larger than normal The presence of macrocytes	
Hypochromic Hypochromia	Paler than normal (more than a third of the diameter of the cell is pale) The presence of hypochromic cells	
Polychromasia	Having a blue tinge	
Elliptocyte	An erythrocyte that is elliptical in shape	

(Continued)

Table 2.4. *(Continued)*

Term	Significance	Picture
Ovalocyte	An erythrocyte that is oval in shape	
Macro-ovalocyte	An oval macrocyte	
Spherocyte	An erythrocyte that is spherical in shape and is therefore lacking central pallor	
Irregularly contracted cell	An erythrocyte that lacks central pallor and has an irregular outline	
Teardrop cell (dacrocyte)	An erythrocyte that is shaped like a tear	

(Continued)

Table 2.4. *(Continued)*

Term	Significance	Picture
Target cell	An erythrocyte that has haemoglobin concentrated at the periphery of the cell and also as a dot in the centre	
Sickle cell	An erythrocyte with a crescent or sickle shape	
Stomatocyte	An erythrocyte with a slit-like 'stoma'	
Schistocyte or fragment	A small piece of a red cell	

(Continued)

Table 2.4.   (*Continued*)

Term	Significance	Picture
Acanthocyte	An erythrocyte that has a small number of spicules of irregular length	
Echinocyte or crenated cell	An erythrocyte that has a large number of short regular spicules	
Rouleaux	Red cells stacked up like a flattened pile of pennies	
Agglutination	Red cells forming irregular clumps	

(*Continued*)

Table 2.4. *(Continued)*

Term	Significance	Picture
Howell–Jolly body	A fragment of the nucleus remaining in a mature red cell (stains purple)	
Pappenheimer body	An iron-containing granule (stains navy blue)	
Basophilic stippling	Fine or coarse dark blue-staining dots scattered through the cytoplasm	

falsely classified as sick, there are no false positives but the test becomes very insensitive (a lot of false negative results). Fortunately, the overlap between healthy and sick is not often as extreme as shown in Fig. 2.3b.

It can be useful to have a 'health-related range', rather than a normal range that represents 95% of the apparently healthy population. For example, if the upper 20% of results for serum cholesterol in a typical Western population indicated an increased risk of myocardial infarction, an individual and his physician might aim to alter his life style and medications so that his results fell in the bottom 80% of the reference range rather than the central 95%. This bottom 80% would be the health-related range.

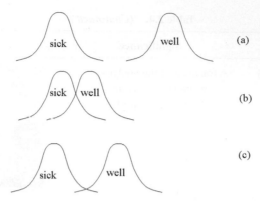

Fig. 2.3. Paired histograms showing the possible results of applying a test in sick and healthy individuals: (a) an ideal test; (b) a non-ideal test that will necessarily result in either false positive or false negative results, depending on the threshold chosen; (c) a test that shows sufficient discrimination between sick and healthy individuals to be useful in clinical practice.

When laboratories collect data to establish a normal range they perform the specified test on healthy volunteers using exactly the same instruments and methods that they are going to use for analysing patient samples. They will also analyse the data using appropriate statistical methods. If the data have a Gaussian distribution, e.g. the Hb (Fig. 2.4), then the arithmetic mean ± two standard deviations (or, more strictly, 1.95 standard deviations) can be used. The WBC, however, has a logarithmic distribution (Fig. 2.5) and the data have to be converted to logarithms before they can be analysed. Other non-Gaussian distributions have to be dealt with by other statistical techniques.

It is important when interpreting laboratory tests to take account of the following: (i) the normal range may not be appropriate; (ii) the test result may be within the normal range but abnormal for that patient; and (iii) the test result might be outside the reference range but actually normal.

Laboratories usually have only two normal ranges, for adult men and for adult women. Normal ranges for children often differ from those for adults, normal ranges for pregnant women differ form those of non-pregnant women (e.g. the Hb is lower and the WBC and MCV are higher) and normal ranges for individuals of African ancestry differ from those of Northern Europeans (the FBC, neutrophil count and platelet count are lower).

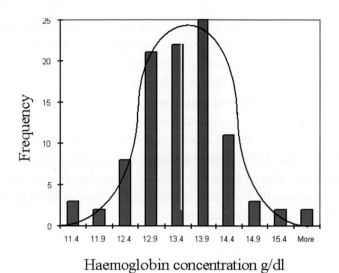

Fig. 2.4. A histogram of Hb results in healthy subjects showing a Gaussian distribution.

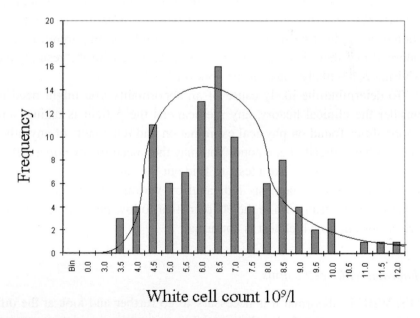

Fig. 2.5. A histogram of WBC results in healthy subjects showing a skewed distribution that will become Gaussian on logarithmic transformation.

A test result for an individual patient may still be within the normal range but nevertheless be abnormal for that individual. For example, a man could have a major gastrointestinal haemorrhage and next day, as a result of haemodilution, his Hb has fallen from his usual level of 16.5 g/dl to 14 g/dl. This is still within the normal range but is very abnormal for him.

If the normal range represents results from 95% of healthy subjects there will always be normal results that fall outside the 'normal' range. This will be so for 5% of results for each test. If a lot of tests are done it is very probable that at least one will be abnormal. For example, if the eight tests that usually form part of the FBC are performed it is likely that a third of patients will have an abnormal result.

How to Interpret a Blood Count and Develop a Differential Diagnosis

When interpreting a blood count, or any other laboratory result, you should ask yourself the following questions: (i) is this result abnormal for this patient?; (ii) if it is abnormal, is it a trivial abnormality that should be ignored or might it be important?; (iii) if it might be important, is it so abnormal that there is a clinical urgency in dealing with the result?; and (iv) what is the likely cause of the abnormality?

To determine the likely cause of an abnormality you might need to consider the clinical history, any medications the patient is taking, any abnormalities found on physical examination and the results of any other tests that have already been done. You may then need to develop a differential diagnosis and do extra tests to find out the cause.

The differential diagnosis indicated by various blood count abnormalities will be dealt with in the chapters that follow but will be outlined here, according to which test is abnormal.

Abnormal white cell counts

If the WBC is abnormal it is necessary to go further and look at the different components of the differential count to see which parts are abnormal. The automated instrument that produces the WBC is likely to have produced an automated differential count. If the abnormality is purely quantitative, e.g. an increased neutrophil count, then the clinical history may reveal the cause (e.g. known bacterial infection) so that no further haematological tests are indicated. On other occasions there may be immature cells present or abnormalities of mature cells so that the automated instrument either does not produce a differential count or 'flags' the result, indicating an abnormality. In this instance a blood film is usually needed.

The neutrophil count

In deciding if a neutrophil count is elevated or reduced it is important to make a comparison with a relevant reference range (e.g. counts are higher in pregnancy and lower in some individuals of African ancestry).

A high neutrophil count is usually reactive to infection, inflammation, trauma or surgery, and is due to increased production by the bone marrow. Rarely, it is due to leukaemia.

A low neutrophil count can be due to: (i) inadequate production by the bone marrow; (ii) inability of the bone marrow to respond sufficiently to increased need, e.g. in infected neonates; (iii) peripheral destruction, e.g. drug-induced immune destruction; or (iv) abnormal pooling, e.g. in the spleen in hypersplenism.

The lymphocyte count

A high lymphocyte count can be due to increased production of lymphocytes or to altered distribution within the body. Increased production can be reactive, e.g. to viral infection, or be the result of leukaemia. A high lymphocyte count due to mobilisation of lymphocytes from tissues occurs as a transient acute response to stress, e.g. following severe trauma or a myocardial infarction. Lymphocytosis due to redistribution of lymphocytes within the body also occurs following splenectomy.

A low lymphocyte count can be due to inherited and acquired immune deficiency, e.g. HIV infection, or can be a stress response to illness, surgery or trauma, in that case being mediated by corticosteroids. A stress-induced lymphocytosis is followed by a stress-induced lymphopenia.

The monocyte count

An increased monocyte count is usually reactive, as the result of chronic infection, inflammation or malignancy and is the result of increased production by the bone marrow. Less often it represents leukaemia.

A reduced monocyte count is usually due to inadequate production by the bone marrow. It is uncommon but when it does occur it renders the patient susceptible to infection.

The eosinophil count

An increased eosinophil count is usually reactive, as a result of allergy (including some adverse drug reactions) or parasitic infection, and is due to increased bone marrow production.

A low eosinophil count occurs as a stress reaction, mediated by corticosteroids.

The basophil count

An increased basophil count is often a feature of a haematological neoplasm and results from increased bone marrow production. It is diagnostically useful since reactive basophilia (e.g. due to hypothyroidism or ulcerative colitis) is uncommon.

A reduced basophil count is rarely noted and is even more rarely of diagnostic importance.

Anaemia

The cause of the anaemia may be apparent from the clinical history. If not, a differential diagnosis can be developed by considering the size of the cells or by trying to work out the mechanism of the anaemia. A classification of anaemia based on cell size is shown in Table 2.5. This approach is very useful and often indicates a likely diagnosis and the tests that are needed to confirm it. If consideration of clinical features and erythrocyte size does not suggest a diagnosis it can be useful to seek evidence of a mechanism of the anaemia, as shown in Table 2.6.

Table 2.5. Classification of anaemias according to cell size.

Cell size	Microcytic	Macrocytic	Normocytic
Causes	Iron deficiency (common) Anaemia of chronic disease (common) Thalassaemia (common in some ethnic groups)	Liver disease Alcohol excess Megaloblastic anaemia (vitamin B_{12} or folate deficiency or exposure to certain drugs) Myelodysplastic syndromes Hypothyroidism Aplastic anaemia Haemolysis	Early stages or iron deficiency and anaemia of chronic disease Blood loss Renal failure Bone marrow suppression (e.g. by chemotherapy)

Table 2.6. Classification of anaemia according to mechanism.

Mechanism	Possible supporting evidence
Failure of bone marrow production	Low reticulocyte count, lack of polychromasia
Blood loss	Clinical evidence and later increased reticulocyte count
Increased destruction (i.e. haemolysis)	Increased reticulocyte count, polychromasia, increased bilirubin concentration, increased lactate dehydrogenase, cells of abnormal shape (spherocytes, elliptocytes, fragments)
Red cell pooling in the spleen plus increased plasma volume	Clinical evidence — presence of splenomegaly

Polycythaemia

Polycythaemia refers to an increase of RBC, Hb and Hct. These laboratory abnormalities can be the result of a true polycythaemia, in which the total volume of red cells circulating in the bloodstream is increased. This can also be the result of an acute or chronic reduction of plasma volume, referred to as pseudopolycythaemia. The cause of an acute reduction in plasma volume, e.g. shock, burns or dehydration, will be apparent from the clinical history but a chronic pseudopolycythaemia requires laboratory tests to distinguish it from true polycythaemia. The differential diagnosis of polycythaemia will be discussed in Chapter 9.

Thrombocytosis

A high platelet count is almost always due to increased production by the bone marrow. The exception is following splenectomy, when it is due to redistribution. Thrombocytosis is usually reactive, due to infection, inflammation, blood loss or malignancy. Less often it is the result of a chronic haematological neoplasm known as a myeloproliferative neoplasm.

Thrombocytopenia can be the result of: (i) failure of bone marrow production; (ii) increased destruction by antibodies; (iii) increased consumption during coagulation; (iii) blood loss with failure to replace platelets that are lost; or (iv) pooling in an enlarged spleen. The causes of thrombocytopenia will be discussed in more detail in Chapter 11.

The Erythrocyte Sedimentation Rate

This test involves mixing blood with the correct amount of citrate anticoagulant, allowing it to sediment in a tube of precise dimensions and measuring the number of mm the red cells have sedimented at the end of one hour. The normal range is 1–10 mm in an hour for a man and 0–20 mm in an hour for a woman. The erythrocyte sedimentation rate (ESR) is increased by anaemia and decreased by polycythaemia. It is increased by an increase in large plasma proteins (such as fibrinogen, $\alpha 2$ macroglobulin and immunoglobulins, particularly immunoglobulin M) and by a reduction in albumin concentration. The ESR is increased by pregnancy and by infection, inflammation, tissue infarction and malignancy. Although this test is very non-specific, it remains useful for monitoring chronic inflammatory conditions, such as rheumatoid arthritis, and in the follow up of Hodgkin lymphoma.

Conclusions

In order to interpret a full blood count and blood film you need to be familiar with the terminology and the abbreviations that are usually used. You also need to know the approximate normal range for common measurements. By the time you get to the end of this book, or your haematology course, you should also be able to interpret a blood count and film, develop a differential diagnosis and explain what tests you would do next.

3

Microcytic Anaemias and the Thalassaemias

What Do You Have to Know?

☞ How to diagnose, investigate and treat iron deficiency anaemia
☞ When to suspect and how to diagnose anaemia of chronic disease
☞ The nature of thalassaemia, how it is diagnosed, why diagnosis is important and how the condition is managed
☞ That there are other causes of microcytic anaemia

Introduction

A microcytic anaemia is one in which the erythrocytes are smaller than normal (i.e. microcytic). Often they also hypochromic (i.e. they appear paler than normal in a stained blood film). The anaemia may thus be referred to as a hypochromic microcytic anaemia. The blood count shows a reduced haemoglobin concentration (Hb), haematocrit (Hct) and mean cell volume (MCV). Cells of reduced size tend to have a reduced haemoglobin content so the mean cell haemoglobin (MCH) is also reduced. In addition, the concentration of haemoglobin in the erythrocytes is reduced; this may be reflected in a low normal value or a reduction in the mean cell haemoglobin concentration (MCHC).

41

Microcytic anaemias result from a reduced rate of synthesis of haemoglobin. This, in turn, results from a reduced rate of synthesis of either **haem**
or **globin**. A reduced rate of synthesis of haem occurs in iron deficiency and
also in a type of anaemia that occurs in patients with chronic infection or
inflammation, known as 'anaemia of chronic disease'. Unlike iron deficiency,
in the anaemia of chronic disease body stores of iron are normal or increased;
however, the availability of iron to the developing red cell is reduced. A
reduced rate of synthesis of either α or β globin chains also leads to a reduced
rate of synthesis of haemoglobin and thus to microcytosis. A reduced rate of
synthesis of one or other of the globin chain types is usually an inherited condition, known as α thalassaemia (reduced rate of α globin chains) or β
thalassaemia (reduced rate of synthesis of β globin chains). A rare cause of a
microcytic anaemia is an inherited defect in the synthesis of haem in which
iron accumulates within the mitochondria of erythroblasts rather than being
incorporated into haem; this is known as sideroblastic anaemia. Rarely
acquired defects in haem synthesis occur, for example in lead poisoning.

The various mechanisms of microcytosis are summarised in Fig. 3.1.

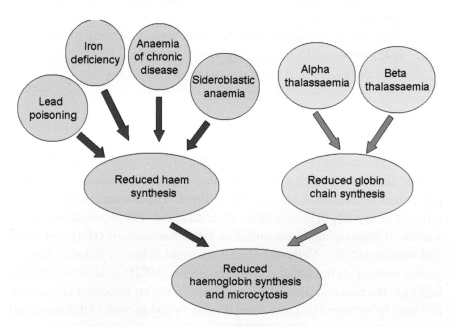

Fig. 3.1.   Diagrammatic representation of the causes of microcytosis.

Iron Deficiency Anaemia

Iron, which is essential for the synthesis of haemoglobin, is obtained from the diet and recycled and conserved in the body. Dietary sources and absorption are discussed on page 12. To maintain a normal Hb, iron absorption needs to keep up with any physiological or pathological loss and cope with any increased demands. Iron deficiency therefore results from: (i) inadequate intake; (ii) malabsorption; (iii) increased need; (iv) increased or abnormal loss; and (v) any combination of these factors (Fig. 3.2, Table 3.1). In developed countries iron deficiency is the most common cause of anaemia, accounting for almost a third of cases. This proportion is even higher in developing countries. Common causes of iron deficiency are poor dietary intake of iron, increased requirements (in infancy or during pregnancy) and abnormal blood loss. In developing countries blood loss from intestinal parasites is a major factor. Low socioeconomic status and poverty correlate with an increased rate of iron deficiency. In infants, early

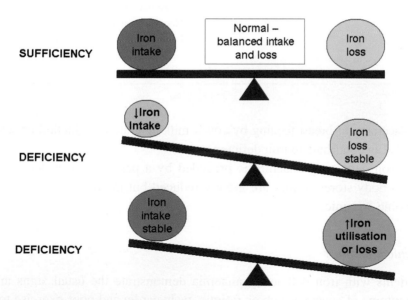

Fig. 3.2. Diagrammatic representation of the causes of iron deficiency: (a) balanced intake and loss, normal iron status (b) decreased iron intake that does not balance iron loss; iron deficiency occurs (c) increased iron utilisation in excess of what is provided by normal intake; iron deficiency occurs.

Table 3.1.   **Factors that can cause or contribute to iron deficiency anaemia.**

Increased utilisation	Inadequate intake	Malabsorption	Increased loss	Sequestration of iron
Growth spurts, e.g. in infants, children and adolescents Repeated pregnancies and lactation	Weaning babies onto iron-poor milk or substitutes (e.g. 'goat's milk anaemia') Vegetarian diet	Coeliac disease Autoimmune gastric atrophy *Helicobacter pylori* infection	Menorrhagia Gastrointestinal bleeding (e.g. induced by aspirin or other non-steroidal anti-inflammatory drugs, other ulceration, inflammatory bowel disease, carcinoma and [in some countries] intestinal parasites) Haemoglobinuria Frequently repeated blood donation	Pulmonary haemosiderosis

replacement of breast feeding by cow's milk and late introduction of solid foods can contribute to iron deficiency.

Iron deficiency anaemia is preceded by a period of iron depletion, when body stores of iron are greatly reduced but the patient has not yet become anaemic.

Clinical features

Patients with iron deficiency anaemia demonstrate the usual signs and symptoms of anaemia such as fatigue, tachycardia and poor exercise tolerance. Specific clinical features suggestive of iron deficiency are uncommon. They include pica (the ingestion of unusual substances such as ice or soil), glossitis (flattening and soreness of the tongue), angular cheilosis (cracking at the angle of the mouth), dysphagia and koilonychia (spoon-shaped nails). In children there may also be impaired intellectual performance, which may not be reversible.

Laboratory features

Iron deficiency anaemia is initially normocytic and normochromic. As it becomes more severe, it become hypochromic and microcytic. The red cell count (RBC), Hb, Hct, MCV and MCH are all reduced. When the anaemia is severe the MCHC is also reduced. The platelet count may be increased. When iron deficiency is the result of intestinal parasites such as hookworm (Fig. 3.3) the blood count may show eosinophilia.

The blood film shows hypochromia and microcytosis (Fig. 3.4). When anaemia is more severe there is anisocytosis and poikilocytosis, with thin

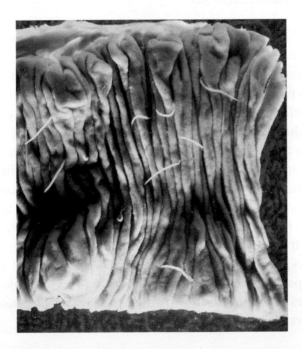

Fig. 3.3. Adult hookworms attached by their buccal capsule to the villi of the small intestine. Hookworm is an important worldwide cause of iron deficiency anaemia. Eosinophilia is maximal at the stage of larval migration through the lung. Reproduced with permission from Peters, W. and Pasvol, G. (2007). *Atlas of Tropical Medicine and Parasitology*, 6th Edn, Elsevier, Philadelphia.

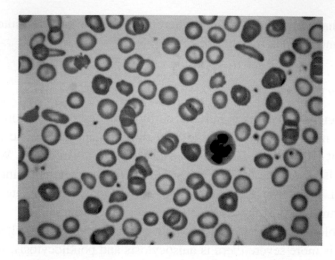

Fig. 3.4. Peripheral blood (PB) film in iron deficiency anaemia showing hypochromia, microcytosis and several elliptocytes.

elliptocytes, known as pencil cells, being particularly characteristic. There may be small numbers of target cells.

Serum ferritin is usually low and as other causes of a low ferritin are very rare a reduced ferritin, e.g. less than 15 μg/l (normal range [NR] 15–300) confirms that anaemia is the result of iron deficiency. Serum iron is low and the transferrin concentration and the iron-binding capacity are elevated but these measurements are not necessary if the ferritin is low.

In patients with chronic inflammation the diagnosis of iron deficiency is more difficult since serum ferritin is elevated by infection, acute and chronic inflammation and many tumours. In patients known to have these conditions a ferritin of up to 50 μg/l or even higher is consistent with iron deficiency. If the results of blood tests do not clearly distinguish between these two types of anaemia a bone marrow aspirate will provide the answer. In patients with iron deficiency, there is no stainable iron in the macrophages of the bone marrow particles whereas in anaemia of chronic disease, storage iron is present and may be increased.

Diagnosis

A blood count, blood film and serum ferritin assay are usually all that is required for diagnosis. In uncomplicated iron deficiency there is a hypochromic microcytic anaemia and a low serum ferritin. When diagnosis is difficult, it may be necessary to examine the bone marrow and perform a Prussian blue stain on a bone marrow film. In a normal bone marrow, iron is present in macrophages within bone marrow fragments and stains deep blue (Fig. 3.5); it is also seen as small blue-staining particles within erythroblasts, referred to as siderotic granules. In iron deficiency no blue-staining material is apparent in the fragments (Fig. 3.6) and siderotic granules are reduced or absent.

Management

Having established a diagnosis of iron deficiency it is necessary both to find the cause and deal with it and to treat the deficiency. Dietary history, travel history and the number and frequency of pregnancies must be assessed. The possibility of menorrhagia or other abnormal bleeding must be considered. In young women low dietary iron intake, menstruation and pregnancy are the likely causes. In middle-aged or elderly people of either gender gastrointestinal tract bleeding (which may be occult) is likely. Other potential causes to consider are malabsorption of iron due to achlorhydria or coeliac disease (serology for anti-tissue transglutaminase antibodies should be performed). Patients with pernicious anaemia (see

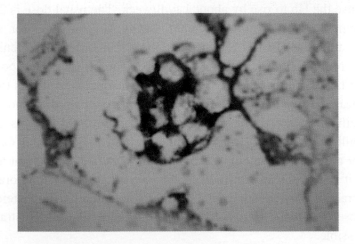

Fig. 3.5. Bone marrow (BM) fragment stained with a Perls' stain for iron showing that storage iron (haemosiderin in macrophages) is present (blue-staining material).

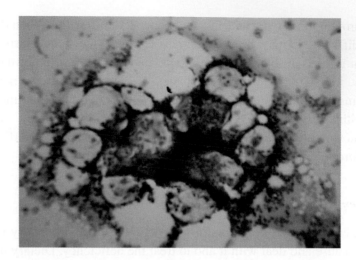

Fig. 3.6. BM stained with a Perls' stain for iron in a patient with iron deficiency anaemia showing that storage iron (haemosiderin in macrophages) is absent (no blue-staining material).

page 69) have achlorhydria and are prone to iron deficiency. In middle-aged and elderly patients (e.g. above 50 years) investigations to exclude gastrointestinal carcinoma or other tumours must be carried out, even in the absence of relevant symptoms.

Iron deficiency is usually treated with oral ferrous sulphate, which will cause the Hb to rise by about 1 g/dl/week. The usual dose is 200 mg three times a day. Treatment should ideally be continued for several months after the Hb has returned to normal in order to replenish the body's iron stores. The patient should be warned that the stools will become black and that there may be gastrointestinal side effects (nausea, diarrhoea, constipation, abdominal pain). Mothers of children should also be specifically warned to keep the iron preparation in a safe place away from children. Accidental iron poisoning in children can be fatal. Oral iron is better absorbed on an empty stomach but if the patient cannot tolerate it then it can be taken with food. If the patient cannot tolerate oral iron, parenteral preparations are available, most conveniently administered as a total dose intravenous infusion although intramuscular administration is also possible.

Anaemia of Chronic Disease

Anaemia of chronic disease, also known as anaemia of inflammation, characteristically occurs in patients with chronic infection or inflammation. It also occurs in some patients with malignant disease. Typical causes include tuberculosis, rheumatoid arthritis, ulcerative colitis, Crohn's disease, carcinoma of the ovary and Hodgkin lymphoma. Anaemia of chronic disease is characterised by iron-deficient erythropoiesis but body stores of iron are normal or increased. The mechanism is synthesis of an inflammatory cytokine, interleukin 6, by macrophages. This stimulates hepcidin synthesis by the liver. The result of a high plasma hepcidin level is that iron is retained in macrophages rather than being released to transferrin for delivery to erythroblasts (Fig. 3.7). Hepcidin also reduces export of iron from enterocytes

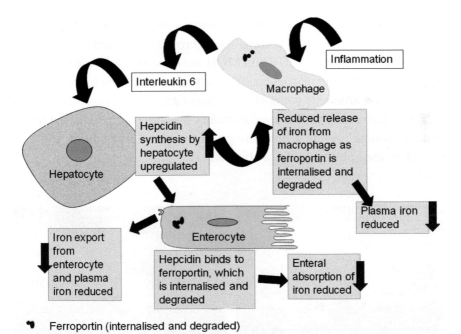

Fig. 3.7. Diagram showing how hepcidin regulates iron absorption and release from macrophages and how increases in interleukin 6 (synthesised by macrophages when there is inflammation) leads to increased hepcidin synthesis and contributes to the anaemia of chronic disease.

to the plasma, again reducing availability of iron. Other mechanisms can contribute to the anaemia of chronic disease, including a blunted erythropoietin response to anaemia and some reduction in red cell life span.

Clinical features

There are no specific clinical features. Usually the primary disease responsible for anaemia of chronic disease is clinically apparent but sometimes the cause is an occult infection or tumour. Anaemia of chronic disease is the second most common cause of anaemia in developed countries, not much behind iron deficiency in frequency.

Laboratory features

Anaemia of chronic disease is initially normocytic and normochromic. As it becomes more severe, it become hypochromic and microcytic. At this stage the RBC, Hb, Hct, MCV and MCH are all reduced. The white blood cell count (WBC) and platelet count may be increased. The blood film initially shows normocytic normochromic and later hypochromic microcytic red cells. There may be increased rouleaux formation and increased background staining (giving a bluish tinge to the blood film), both resulting from increased plasma proteins (Fig. 3.8).

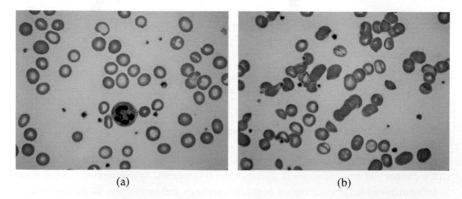

(a)   (b)

Fig. 3.8.   PB in anaemia of chronic disease in a patient with rheumatoid arthritis showing (a) hypochromia and microcytosis and (b) some increase in rouleaux formation.

Serum ferritin is elevated. Serum iron is reduced but, in contrast to iron deficiency anaemia, serum transferrin and iron-binding capacity are also reduced. There may be an increased erythrocyte sedimentation rate (ESR) and increased C-reactive protein, $\alpha2$ macroglobulin, fibrinogen and immunoglobulins. The usual test results in comparison with those in iron deficiency are shown in Table 3.2. In most patients with anaemia of chronic disease, examination of the bone marrow shows normal or increased iron stores but siderotic granules are reduced as iron is not being delivered to the developing erythroblasts.

However, many of the conditions that can cause anaemia of chronic disease can also lead, directly or indirectly, to iron deficiency. Inflammatory bowel disease can lead to gastrointestinal blood loss as can the drugs used for treatment of rheumatoid arthritis (aspirin and non-steroidal anti-inflammatory drugs). When anaemia of chronic disease

Table 3.2. **Blood tests in iron deficiency anaemia and the anaemia of chronic disease.**

	Iron deficiency anaemia	Anaemia of chronic disease	Normal range Men	Normal range Women
Serum ferritin	↓	Normal or ↑	15–300 µg/l	15–200 µg/l
Serum iron	↓	↓	12–24 µmol/l	9–23 µmol/l
Serum transferrin	↑	Normal or ↓	1.7–3.4 g/l	
Iron-binding capacity			54–72 µmol/l	55–81 µmol/l
Transferrin saturation	↓	↓	18–40%	13–37%
Soluble transferrin receptor*	↑ (e.g. >2.3 mg/l)	Normal or slightly ↑ (e.g. <2.3 mg/l)	0.85–3.06 mg/l*	
Soluble transferrin receptor* / Log ferritin	>1.36 (or >1.5)	<1.36 (or <1.5)	≤1.36 (or ≤1.5)*	
C-reactive protein	Normal	↑	<5 mg/l	
Erythrocyte sedimentation rate	Normal or near normal	↑	1–10 mm in 1 hour	1–20 mm in 1 hour
Bone marrow storage iron	Absent	Normal or ↑	Present	Usually present

* Very dependent on method of measurement of soluble transferrin receptor.

co-exists with iron deficiency, results of laboratory tests may be equivocal and sometimes a bone marrow aspirate is necessary to demonstrate that there is absent bone marrow iron.

Management

Effective management of the primary disease will lead to improvement of the anaemia. Other types of therapy that are sometimes used include erythropoietin injections and blood transfusion.

The Thalassaemias

To understand the thalassaemias, it is necessary to know which haemoglobins are normally present in the fetus, baby and adult (Table 3.3) and to understand the basics of the genetic control of globin chain synthesis. A normal fetus has mainly fetal haemoglobin (haemoglobin F) but, before birth, synthesis of adult haemoglobin (haemoglobin A) commences and steadily

Table 3.3. **Haemoglobins present at various stages of life.**

Haemoglobin	Constituent chains	When present	Genes needed	Proportion in adult
F (fetal haemoglobin)	$\alpha_2\gamma_2$	Fetal life and early neonatal period; minor component in child and adult	α $^G\gamma$, $^A\gamma$ or both	Less than 1%
A (adult hemoglobin)	$\alpha_2\beta_2$	Late fetal life and increasingly major proportion in neonate, infant, child and adult	α β	95.5–97.5%
A_2	$\alpha_2\delta_2$	Increases from neonatal period onwards but always very minor component	α δ	2.0–3.5%

increases as haemoglobin F synthesis decreases (Fig. 3.9). Haemoglobin A_2 synthesis starts later than synthesis of haemoglobin A; it is always a minor component but is diagnostically important. The α globin chains are encoded by a pair of α genes ($\alpha2$ and $\alpha1$) in the α gene cluster on each chromosome 16. The γ, β and δ chains are encoded by γ, β and δ genes in the β cluster on each chromosome 11.

The thalassaemias are a group of inherited disorders in which a mutation or deletion of a gene encoding one of the globin chains results in a reduced rate of synthesis, or absent synthesis, of the equivalent chain. This leads to a reduced rate of synthesis of haemoglobin and therefore microcytosis. In the milder forms of thalassaemia (often referred to as thalassaemia trait), the bone marrow can compensate by producing more red cells so that there is microcytosis without anaemia. In the more severe forms of thalassaemia there is anaemia and, in the most severe forms, either this is fatal or life is sustained only by regular blood transfusion.

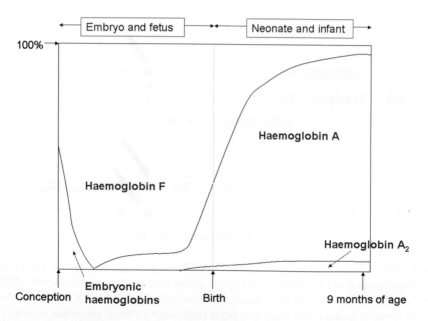

Fig. 3.9. The proportions of various haemoglobins present in intrauterine life and in neonates and young infants.

β *thalassaemias*

Normal cells have two β globin genes. β thalassaemia is a condition resulting from mutation in one or both of the β globin genes (Fig. 3.10), which leads to a reduced rate, or even a total absence, of synthesis of β globin. β thalassaemia genes are highly prevalent in many parts of the world: about 15% in Cyprus, up to 20% in some parts of Italy, Greece and Turkey; 5–10% in South-East Asia; about 5% overall in the Indian sub-continent; and about 1% in Afro-Caribbeans.

β *thalassaemia heterozygosity*

If there is a mutation in only one of the two β globin genes there is a reduced rate of synthesis of β globin and therefore microcytosis. However,

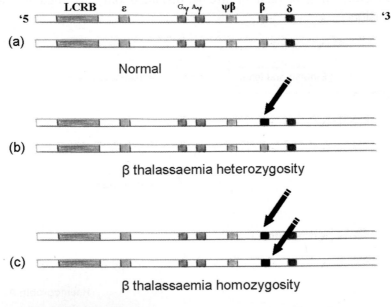

Fig. 3.10.   Diagram of the β globin gene cluster showing the γ, β and δ genes. ε is a gene that operates only in embryonic life and ψβ is a pseudogene (i.e. it is non-functional). LCRB indicates a master control of these genes, the locus control region beta. A normal β globin gene cluster is shown in (a); in (b) a mutation (indicated by a black arrow) has occurred in one β gene, leading to heterozygosity for β thalassaemia, also known as β thalassaemia trait; in (c) a mutation has occurred in both β globin genes, leading to homozygosity for β thalassaemia or, if the two mutations are different, to compound heterozygosity for β thalassaemia.

the bone marrow compensates by producing more red cells so that the blood count usually shows an increased RBC, normal Hb and Hct, and reduced MCV and MCH. These red cell indices are quite different from those of iron deficiency, in which a fall of Hb precedes the development of microcytosis (low MCV and MCH). The MCHC, which can be low in iron deficiency, is typically normal. The blood film may show only microcytosis or there may also be poikilocytes including target cells (Fig. 3.11).

β thalassaemia trait is an asymptomatic condition. Only occasionally, e.g. during pregnancy or intercurrent infection, does anaemia occur. The importance is genetic. If a child inherits a β thalassaemia gene from each parent the result is usually a clinically severe condition known as β thalassaemia major (Fig. 3.12). For this reason doctors should test for β thalassaemia heterozygosity in pregnancy (or preconceptually) and if this is found to be present the partner should also be tested so that, if a fetus is found to be homozygous for β thalassaemia, termination of pregnancy can be offered.

Diagnosis of β thalassaemia heterozygosity is based on the presence of microcytosis plus an elevated proportion of haemoglobin A_2 (measured by high-performance liquid chromatography or microcolumn chromatography). The elevation percentage of this usually minor haemoglobin occurs

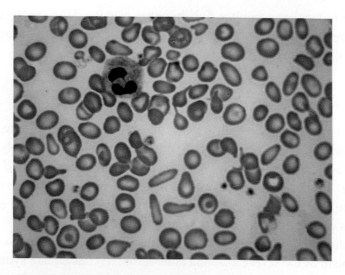

Fig. 3.11. PB film in β thalassaemia heterozygosity showing microcytosis, occasional hypochromic cells, elliptocytes, target cells and other poikilocytes.

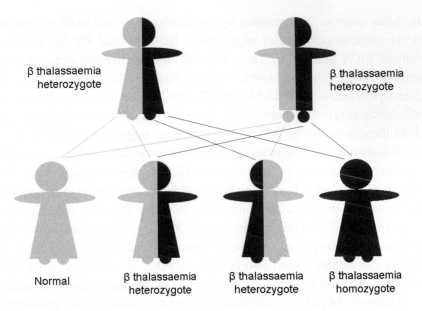

β thalassaemia heterozygote

β thalassaemia heterozygote

Normal

β thalassaemia heterozygote

β thalassaemia heterozygote

β thalassaemia homozygote

Fig. 3.12. The inheritance of β thalassaemia. Both parents have β thalassaemia heterozygosity. For each pregnancy that occurs, there is a one in two chance of β thalassaemia heterozygosity, a one in four chance of normal globin genes and a one in four chance of β thalassaemia major.

because its synthesis requires δ chain rather than the deficient β chain. For similar reasons there is often an increase in the percentage of haemoglobin F since this requires γ chains rather than the deficient β chains.

β thalassaemia homozygosity or compound heterozygosity

If there is a mutation in both β genes the situation is much more serious than when only one is mutated. Synthesis of β globin is totally absent (β^0 thalassaemia) or severely reduced ($\beta^0\beta^+$ thalassaemia or $\beta^+\beta^+$ thalassaemia). This leads to β thalassaemia major, a condition in which survival for more than a few years is dependent on blood transfusion. Failure to thrive is noted between 3 and 6 months of age as haemoglobin F synthesis declines but haemoglobin A synthesis does not take over. The mechanism of the severe anaemia is threefold: (i) inadequate synthesis of globin and therefore of haemoglobin leading to a microcytic anaemia;

(ii) ineffective haemopoiesis — death of red cell precursors in the bone marrow when they are damaged by excess α chains; and (iii) shortened red cell survival. The severe anaemia leads to increased erythropoietin synthesis, which stimulates a further increase in largely ineffective erythropoiesis. This occurs within an expanded bone marrow space (leading to bony deformity) and at extramedullary sites (leading to gross hepatosplenomegaly; Fig. 3.13). The splenomegaly further aggravates the anaemia as red cells are pooled in the spleen.

In countries in which economic circumstances permit, β thalassaemia major is treated by regular blood transfusion. This prevents death from thalassaemia but instead leads to iron overload, with deposition of iron in the heart, pancreas, pituitary and liver. Tissue damage from iron overload leads to death (usually in early adult life from cardiac failure) if iron is not

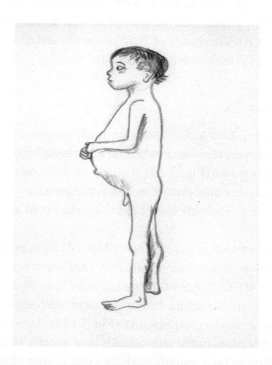

Fig. 3.13. A drawing of a child with β thalassaemia major who has been receiving inadequate transfusion support. He has skull expansion with frontal bossing, expanded maxillae and mandible, gross hepatosplenomegaly (note eversion of the umbilicus) and wasting of his limbs.

removed by chelation. Chelation therapy can be by subcutaneous infusion of desferrioxamine (also known as deferoxamine), which is usually given overnight on 5 nights a week, or by daily oral deferasirox or deferiprone. Bone marrow transplantation should be considered in younger patients who do not yet have serious organ damage from iron overload.

β thalassaemia intermedia

The term 'β thalassaemia intermedia' refers to a genetically heterogeneous group of conditions that range from mildly to severely symptomatic. By definition, survival without blood transfusion is possible although, in the more severe forms, quality of life may be poor in the absence of transfusion. β thalassaemia intermedia can result from heterozygosity for β thalassaemia with aggravating factors or from inheritance of two β thalassaemia genes but with ameliorating factors. In South-East Asia, co-inheritance of β thalassaemia and haemoglobin E is a common cause of β thalassaemia intermedia.

α thalassaemias

Normal cells have two alpha genes on each chromosome 16. Various α thalassaemia syndromes occur when there is deletion or loss of function of 1, 2, 3 or 4 α genes (Fig. 3.14). Usually α thalassaemia results from α gene deletion rather than mutation. The consequences of α gene loss are shown in Table 3.4. The only important things to know are:

1. Loss of one or two α genes (Fig. 3.14b,c,d) can cause microcytosis but is harmless to the individual. It is very common in some ethnic groups (e.g. 25% of Afro-Caribbeans have loss of a single α gene, known as α^+ thalassaemia heterozygosity). Although loss of two α genes from a single chromosome (Fig 3.14d), known as α^0 thalassaemia, is harmless to the individual it is of genetic significance since this condition in both parents leads to a one in four chance of haemoglobin Bart's hydrops fetalis (see below). Diagnosis is by DNA analysis in individuals with microcytosis who are of relevant ethnic origin (South-East Asian, Greek, Cypriot, Turkish or Sardinian).

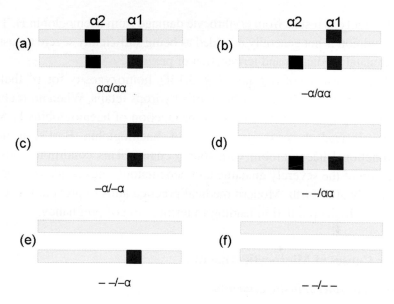

Fig. 3.14. Diagram of normal and abnormal α globin genes: (a) normal, two α genes on each chromosome 16; (b) deletion of a single α gene (α^+ thalassaemia heterozygosity); (c) deletion of a single α gene from each chromosome (α^+ thalassaemia homozygosity); (d) deletion of both α genes from a single chromosome (α^0 thalassaemia heterozygosity); (e) deletion of one α gene from one chromosome 16 and both α genes form the other (haemoglobin H disease); (f) loss of all four α genes (haemoglobin Bart's hydrops fetalis).

Table 3.4. Consequences of loss of one or more α genes.

Alpha genes	Consequences
$\alpha\,\alpha/\alpha\,\alpha$	Normal
$-\,\alpha/\alpha\,\alpha$	Haematologically normal or mild microcytosis
$-\,\alpha/-\,\alpha$	Microcytosis, no clinical or genetic significance
$-\,-/\alpha\,\alpha$	Microcytosis, no clinical significance but is genetically significant
$-\,\alpha/-\,-$	Haemoglobin H disease
$-\,-/-\,-$	Haemoglobin Bart's hydrops fetalis

2. Loss of three α genes (Fig. 3.14e) causes haemoglobin H disease, a condition in which there is a moderately severe microcytic anaemia with haemolysis and splenomegaly. Haemoglobin H is a non-functional haemoglobin with four β chains, formed because of the lack of α chains.

Haemolysis results from erythrocyte damage from haemoglobin H. This condition is not generally regarded as being sufficiently severe to justify prenatal prediction and termination of pregnancy.

3. A total absence of α genes (Fig. 3.14f), homozygosity for α^0 thalassaemia, leads to haemoglobin Bart's hydrops fetalis. When no α chain can be produced there can be no production of haemoglobins F, A or A_2. Instead there is production of haemoglobin Bart's, a nonfunctional haemoglobin with four γ chains. This condition leads to death of the severely anaemic and oedematous fetus *in utero* or death shortly after birth. Modern medical practice aims to prevent this condition by its prediction leading to termination of pregnancy.

Other Causes of Microcytic Anaemia

Congenital sideroblastic anaemia

Congenital sideroblastic anaemia is a rare X-linked condition, in which an inherited defect in haem synthesis causes a microcytic anaemia. The distinctive feature is that the blood film is dimorphic, i.e. there is a population of hypochromic microcytic cells and a population of normal cells (Fig. 3.15).

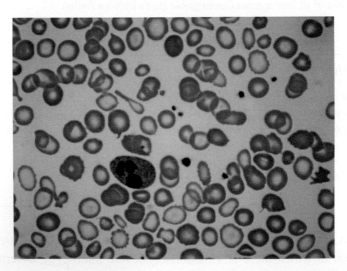

Fig. 3.15. PB film in congenital sideroblastic anaemia showing a dimorphic film: hypochromic microcytic cells and normocytic normochromic cells. There is also anisocytosis and poikilocytosis.

Lead poisoning

Lead poisoning can cause an acquired defect in haem synthesis leading to a microcytic anaemia and can also lead to haemolysis with an increased reticulocyte count. The most distinctive blood film feature is basophilic stippling (Fig. 3.16). Lead poisoning is very rare in developed countries.

Haemoglobinopathies

The presence of a structural variant of haemoglobin is known as a haemo-globinopathy. Often this term also encompasses the thalassaemias. Some haemoglobinopathies are associated with microcytosis.

Haemoglobin E heterozygosity (common in South-East Asia) is usu-ally associated with microcytosis whereas haemoglobin E homozygosity is usually associated with a microcytic anaemia. Haemoglobin C homozy-gosity (found in those of West African ancestry) is associated with a microcytic anaemia.

Conclusions

When a microcytic anaemia is identified, the age, gender, ethnic origin and geographic origin of the patient should be considered. It is also nec-essary to assess the diet, and whether or not there are clinical features to

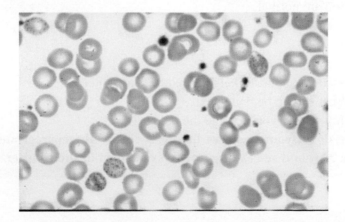

Fig. 3.16. PB film in lead poisoning showing hypochromia and basophilic stippling.

suggest blood loss or chronic infection or inflammation. This information permits a differential diagnosis and the necessary tests to identify iron deficiency, anaemia of chronic disease and other causes of microcytosis can then be requested. If a diagnosis of iron deficiency has been made, it is important to identify the cause. In a patient found to have microcytosis without anaemia, a diagnosis of 'thalassaemia trait' is likely. In these circumstances the ethnic origin should be assessed and the haemoglobin A_2 percentage should be measured; in individuals of child-bearing age of an appropriate ethnic origin, the possibility of α^0 thalassaemia heterozygosity should be considered.

Test Case 3.1

A 63-year-old retired truck driver presents to his general practitioner complaining of fatigue. He has a past history of hypertension and a myocardial infarction and is now taking a β blocker and aspirin, 75 mg daily. A year previously he had suffered from an ill-defined arthritis, which is not currently troubling him. Other than pallor, no abnormality is found on physical examination so some blood tests are done. These show Hb 9 g/dl (normal range [NR] 13.3–16.7) and MCV 75 fl (NR 82–98). The WBC and platelet count are normal. The erythrocyte sedimentation rate is 12 mm in 1 hour (NR < 10) and C-reactive protein (CRP) is 5.5 mg/l (NR < 5). Liver and renal function are normal.

Questions

1. What is the most likely cause of the anaemia?
2. What should be done next?
3. How would you manage the patient?

Write down your answers before checking the correct answer (page 323) and re-reading any relevant part of the chapter.

4

Macrocytic Anaemias

What Do You Have to Know?

☞ The causes of macrocytosis and macrocytic anaemia
☞ How to diagnose, investigate and treat vitamin B_{12} and folate deficiency
☞ When to suspect other causes of macrocytosis

Introduction

A macrocytic anaemia is one in which the average red cell size is greater than normal. The blood count shows an increased mean cell volume (MCV). Macrocytosis can also occur without anaemia. To decide if erythrocytes are larger than normal it is necessary to compare their size with what is normal for an individual of that age, and to compare the MCV of the patient with an appropriate normal range. For example, healthy newborn babies have much larger red cells than children or adults and their erythrocytes would only be considered macrocytic if the MCV was above a normal range for neonates.

Macrocytosis occurs for many reasons (Table 4.1). If there is a deficiency of vitamin B_{12} or folic acid there will be an interference with synthesis of deoxyribonucleic acid (DNA) so that the development of the nucleus is retarded in relation to the maturation of the cytoplasm. The erythroblast continues to grow but cell division is delayed. These large

Table 4.1. Some causes of macrocytosis and macrocytic anaemia.

Classification	Causes
Megaloblastic anaemia	Deficiency of vitamin B_{12} or folic acid
	Drugs interfering with the action of vitamin B_{12} or folic acid and inactivation of vitamin B_{12} by repeated exposure to nitrous oxide (N_2O)
	Other defects in DNA synthesis, e.g. drug-induced and rare congenital defects in pyrimidine synthesis or metabolism of vitamin B_{12} or folic acid
	Some congenital dyserythropoietic anaemias
	Some erythroid leukaemias and myelodysplastic syndromes
Macrocytic anaemia with normoblastic erythropoiesis	Liver disease
	Ethanol toxicity
	Hypothyroidism
	Some myelodysplastic syndromes
	Some congenital dyserythropoietic anaemias
	Some cases of aplastic anaemia
	Some cases of multiple myeloma
	Chronic hypoxic lung disease
'Stress erythropoiesis'	Haemolytic anaemia
	Recovery from anaemia or blood loss

erythroblasts with nucleocytoplasmic dissociation are referred to as megaloblasts (in contrast to erythroblasts without these features, which are known as normoblasts). This type of erythropoiesis is called megaloblastic. In megaloblastic anaemia due to deficiency of vitamin B_{12} or folic acid, the red cell life span is reduced by 30–50%. However, the major cause of the anaemia is ineffective haemopoiesis; this term means that the bone marrow is very cellular but many haemopoietic cells are dying in the bone marrow rather than maturing. Drugs that act as antagonists to vitamin B_{12} (e.g. the anaesthetic agent, nitrous oxide) or folic acid (e.g. methotrexate) also cause a megaloblastic anaemia. Other drugs interfere with DNA synthesis and can cause megaloblastic anaemia. Important among these are: (i) the antiretroviral drug, zidovudine; (ii) the immunosuppressive agent, azathioprine; and (iii) a number of anti-cancer chemotherapeutic agents. There can also be retarded DNA synthesis when the erythroblasts are neoplastic cells, arising from a haemopoietic stem cell that has undergone mutation. This occurs sometimes in acute leukaemias, particularly erythroleukaemias where a large proportion of the leukaemic cells are or erythroid lineage, and also in the myelodysplastic syndromes, which are neoplastic preleukaemic conditions.

In a second major group of macrocytic anaemias the normal relationship between the development of the nucleus and of the cytoplasm is retained but the erythroblasts are larger than normal and so are the resulting red cells. This can be referred to as macronormoblastic erythropoiesis. It occurs in liver disease, as a toxic effect of alcohol and, less often, in hypothyroidism. It also occurs in some myelodysplastic syndromes.

Macrocytosis and macrocytic anaemia can also result from reticulocytosis due to a markedly shortened red cell life span or during the recovery phase after rapid blood loss. A high level of erythropoietin leads to expanded and accelerated erythropoiesis, which is macronormoblastic, and is sometimes called 'stress erythropoiesis.' The circulating red cells include an increased proportion of reticulocytes and other young red cells, which are larger than older red cells. The blood film shows polychromatic macrocytes, representing reticulocytes; some of these have skipped a cell division during erythropoiesis so they can be very large.

Vitamin B_{12} Deficiency

Dietary sources, absorption and function of vitamin B_{12} are discussed on page 15. The causes of vitamin B_{12} deficiency are summarised in Table 4.2.

Table 4.2.   Some of the causes of vitamin B_{12} deficiency.

Nature of cause	Examples
Dietary deficiency	Veganism; a vegetarian diet can contribute to deficiency but does not alone cause tissue deficiency
Gastric causes	Pernicious anaemia, food-B_{12} malabsorption, gastric atrophy associated with *Helicobacter pylori* infection, total or partial gastrectomy, bariatric surgery
Pancreatic causes	Pancreatic insufficiency
Small bowel causes	Coeliac disease, Crohn's disease (particularly after ileal resection), blind loop syndrome, tropical sprue

Anaemia due to vitamin B_{12} (cobalamin) deficiency is much less common than that due to iron deficiency or the anaemia of chronic disease. The most prominent cause in clinical practice is pernicious anaemia (see below). Malabsorption of food-B_{12} (attributed to declining levels of gastric HCl and pepsin with increasing age, possibly aggravated by intake of proton-pump inhibitors) with preserved absorption of crystalline B_{12} is actually more common than pernicious anaemia but usually causes milder, often subclinical, deficiency.

Clinical features

Patients with vitamin B_{12} deficiency may be discovered to have macrocytosis without anaemia or may present with clinical features of anaemia or with neurological complications. There may also be mild jaundice and glossitis. Recognised neurological features include peripheral neuropathy, subacute combined degeneration of the spinal cord, dementia, psychiatric manifestations and optic atrophy. Subacute combined degeneration of the spinal cord involves the dorsal and the corticospinal tracts of the lateral columns resulting in spastic paresis, a Babinski response and reduced proprioception and vibration sense. It should be noted that patients who present with neurological manifestations of vitamin B_{12} deficiency sometime have only a mild macrocytosis and no anaemia.

Laboratory features

Early in the development of vitamin B_{12} deficiency there is usually macrocytosis without anaemia. Later there is a macrocytic anaemia and, when deficiency is very severe, neutropenia and thrombocytopenia. A blood film shows anisocytosis and poikilocytosis with macrocytes, oval macrocytes and hypersegmented neutrophils (six or more nuclear lobes; Fig. 4.1). The absolute reticulocyte count may be reduced, normal or slightly elevated but is inappropriately low for the degree of anaemia. Biochemical tests show increased bilirubin and lactate dehydrogenase and usually increased iron and ferritin. Serum B_{12} is reduced. A bone marrow aspirate shows megaloblastic erythropoiesis and giant metamyelocytes (Figs. 4.2 and 4.3).

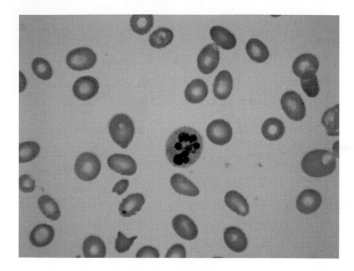

Fig. 4.1. Peripheral blood (PB) film in megaloblastic anaemia showing anisocytosis, macrocytosis, oval macrocytes, a teardrop poikilocyte and a hypersegmented neutrophil.

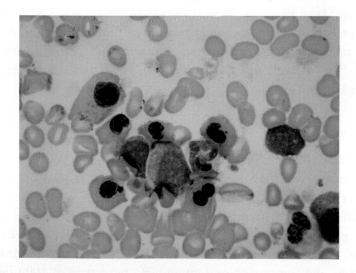

Fig. 4.2. Bone marrow film in severe megaloblastic anaemia. The late erythroblasts show marked megaloblastosis with abundant mature cytoplasm but immature nuclei. Dyserythropoiesis, which is a feature of the megaloblastosis, is present (nuclear lobulation in erythroblasts).

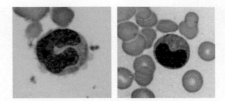

Fig. 4.3. A giant metamyelocyte in the bone marrow in megaloblastic anaemia (left) in comparison with a normal-sized metamyelocyte (right).

Haematological abnormalities may be very mild in those who present with neurological features.

Diagnosis

Diagnosis is based on a blood count, blood film and serum vitamin B_{12} assay. However, it should be noted that many elderly people have a low serum B_{12} without any evidence of tissue deficiency. Conversely, the B_{12} assay is normal in a small minority of patients with confirmed deficiency (less than 5% of patients). If the B_{12} assay is normal when B_{12} deficiency appears otherwise likely, the patient should be further investigated, e.g. by a bone marrow aspirate and by tests relevant to pernicious anaemia (see below). The red cell folate is reduced in about 60% of patients with vitamin B_{12} deficiency.

Management

Treatment is usually with parenteral vitamin B_{12}, in the UK in the form of hydroxocobalamin. Initially 1000 μg can be given at fairly short intervals, e.g. three times a week for 2 weeks, to build up body stores. The mainte-nance dose is then 1000 μg each 3 months. It is customary to give a higher dose in patients with neurological abnormalities but there is no evidence that this is of more benefit than a standard dose. It is also possible to treat vitamin B_{12} deficiency with oral vitamin B_{12} but a dose of 1000 μg a day is needed; absorption is better if not taken with food. Unless a patient has had an allergic reaction to parenteral B_{12} there is no clear advantage to oral therapy.

If vitamin B_{12} deficiency is due to veganism, supplementation of the diet with physiological doses of oral B_{12} is sufficient for maintenance of normality once body stores have been built up.

Management of the patient also requires investigation to establish the cause of the B_{12} deficiency, with treatment of the underlying disease if necessary. The patient's clinical history may indicate a likely diagnosis. Otherwise, investigations are directed mainly at identifying pernicious anaemia, food-B_{12} malabsorption and diseases of the small intestine.

Pernicious anaemia

Pernicious anaemia is an autoimmune disease in which gastric atrophy leads to loss of secretion of pepsin, acid and intrinsic factor with resultant vitamin B_{12} deficiency. There is an association with other autoimmune diseases, such as Addison's disease, hypothyroidism and vitiligo, and there may also be a family history of pernicious anaemia. Autoantibodies directed at gastric parietal cells are present in about 95% of patients and autoantibodies against intrinsic factor in about 60%.

The clinical, haematological and biochemical features are as for any patient with B_{12} deficiency. The diagnosis is most simply made by investigation for intrinsic factor antibodies which, if present, are sufficient to confirm the diagnosis. Investigation for parietal cell antibodies is much less useful since such antibodies are common in elderly people. If intrinsic factor antibodies are not detected (about 30–40% of patients), and if reagents are available, a Schilling test should be performed. The principle of this test is that oral radiolabelled vitamin B_{12} is administered following saturation of B_{12}-binding proteins in the plasma by the administration of non-labelled vitamin B_{12}. The urine is then collected for 24 hours and its radioactivity is measured. Clearly any radiolabelled B_{12} that is excreted must first have been absorbed. If B_{12} excretion is reduced, the test is repeated with intrinsic factor being co-administered with the radiolabelled B_{12}. If the diagnosis is pernicious anaemia there is usually correction of absorption when intrinsic factor is added (Table 4.3).

Management is as for other patients with B_{12} deficiency. Because gastric atrophy also reduces iron absorption some patients with pernicious anaemia have co-existing iron deficiency at presentation and in others the

Table 4.3.   Results expected for the Schilling test with different causes of vitamin B$_{12}$ deficiency.*

Diagnosis	B$_{12}$ administered alone	B$_{12}$ administered with intrinsic factor
Pernicious anaemia	Reduced	Improved
Small bowel malabsorption	Reduced	Not improved
Food-B$_{12}$ malabsorption	Normal	Normal

* It is currently not possible to perform a traditional Schilling test in the UK because of a lack of reagents. It is likely that an alternative test will be developed.

inadequacy of iron stores is revealed by the development of iron deficiency once a haematological response to B$_{12}$ is occurring. Oral iron therapy may then be needed.

It is important to establish a definite diagnosis in pernicious anaemia since patients require life-long therapy.

Folic Acid Deficiency

Dietary sources, absorption and function of folic acid are discussed on page 17. The causes of folic acid deficiency are summarised in Table 4.4. The most common causes are decreased intake and increased requirements.

Clinical features

Patients with folic deficiency have clinical features resulting from anaemia and ineffective erythropoiesis (fatigue, pallor, dyspnoea, mild jaundice).

Laboratory features

The haematological features are usually the same as those of vitamin B$_{12}$ deficiency. However, one of the possible causes of folate deficiency is an increased need for the vitamin so that occasionally the features of a haemolytic anaemia (e.g. hereditary spherocytosis, autoimmune

Table 4.4. Some causes of folic acid deficiency.*

Increased need	Decreased availability	Interference with metabolism	Increased loss
Pregnancy	Reduced dietary	Inborn errors of	Increased urinary
Lactation	intake (poverty,	metabolism	loss (congestive
Prematurity	old age, alcoholism,	Anti-folate drugs	cardiac failure,
Growth spurts	ill-advised diets,	(methotrexate,	active liver
Alcoholism	e.g. 'goat's milk	pyrimethamine,	damage) or
Increased cell	anaemia')	trimethoprim)	other loss
turnover (e.g.	Decreased absorption		(haemodialysis
haemolytic	(coeliac disease,		or peritoneal
anaemia,	jejunal resection,		dialysis)
psoriasis,	tropical sprue,		
chronic	malabsorption		
exfoliative	induced by drugs —		
dermatitis,	sulphasalazine,		
leukaemia)	cholestyramine,		
	triamterine)		

* In addition, folate deficiency appears to be sometimes the result of use of other drugs including phenytoin, primidone and barbiturates.

Table 4.5. Methylmalonic acid and homocysteine assays in deficiency of Vitamin B_{12} and folic acid.

	Methylmalonic acid*	Homocysteine*
Vitamin B_{12} deficiency	↑	↑
Folic acid deficiency	Normal	↑

* Also increased in renal insufficiency.

haemolytic anaemia or sickle cell anaemia) are combined with the features of a megaloblastic anaemia. The serum folate and red cell folate are usually low. Serum B_{12} is reduced in up to a third of patients. Serum bilirubin and LDH are increased. Although not widely available, assays of serum methylmalonic acid and homocysteine can help to distinguish between deficiency of vitamin B_{12} and of folic acid (Table 4.5).

Diagnosis

Assay of red cell folate is the preferred test for diagnosis since it reflects body stores of folate during the previous 2–3 months. Serum folate is more sensitive but is much less specific than red cell folate since serum folate falls within days of a reduction in intake. It is essential to measure serum vitamin B_{12} also since the red cell folate is low in 50% of patients with B_{12} deficiency. Treating B_{12}-deficient patients with pharmacological doses of folic acid will correct the megaloblastic anaemia but permits the neurological defects to progress.

It should be noted that red cell folate may not be low if megaloblastic anaemia develops very acutely. It is therefore important to interpret the laboratory tests in the light of the clinical features.

Management

Treatment is with oral folic acid in a dose of 1–5 mg daily. Management also includes ascertaining the cause of the folic acid deficiency so that the patient can be given dietary advice and conditions such as coeliac disease can be treated.

In patients prone to develop folic acid deficiency, e.g. those with a chronic haemolytic anaemia, folic acid supplementation, e.g. 5 mg a day, is usually given. It is also important to prevent subclinical folate deficiency in women who are, or who might become, pregnant since even sub-clinical deficiency can cause defects in neural tube closure in the fetus leading to spinal bifida. In some countries (e.g. Canada and the United States) this is achieved by supplementing the flour that is used for bread making. In countries where this is not the practice, it is desirable to supplement the normal dietary intake with a further 400 μg of folic acid daily, preferably starting before conception.

Other Causes of Macrocytosis

Macrocytosis is common in the myelodysplastic syndromes, as a result of the dysplastic erythropoiesis (Fig. 4.4). These syndromes will be discussed further in Chapter 6.

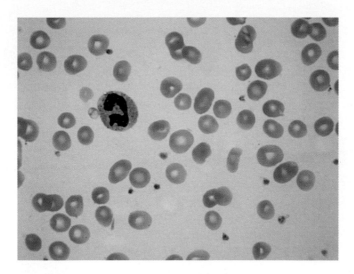

Fig. 4.4. PB film of a patient with refractory anaemia, a form of myelodysplastic syndrome, showing mild anisocytosis and the presence of some macrocytes.

In Western countries excess alcohol intake is probably the most frequent cause of macrocytosis, often with mild anaemia and thrombocytopenia (Fig. 4.5). The mechanism is complex. There may be poor dietary intake of folate and alcohol has a weak antifolate effect; when this is the mechanism there will be megaloblastosis. In other patients there is macronormoblastic erythropoiesis and no biochemical evidence of folate deficiency. When excess alcohol intake is the cause of macrocytosis, the blood film may also show stomatocytosis (Fig. 4.6).

Macrocytosis is also common in liver disease that is not due to alcohol. In these patients there may also be target cells. When there is obstructive jaundice target cells can be very numerous (Fig. 4.7).

Erythrocytes become smaller as they age. Therefore, when there is a chronic haemolytic anaemia the younger red cell population is composed, on average, of larger red cells than when the red cell population shows a normal spread of cell ages. This is most marked when the reticulocyte count is high as reticulocytes are considerable larger than other erythrocytes. The presence of polychromatic macrocytes is a clue to reticulocytosis as a cause of macrocytosis (Fig. 4.8).

74

Chapter 4

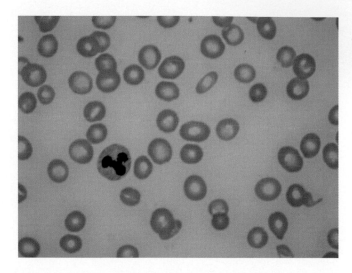

Fig. 4.5. PB film from a patient taking excess alcohol showing anaemia, anisocytosis and macrocytosis. Note that, in contrast to megaloblastic anaemia, the neutrophil is normally segmented.

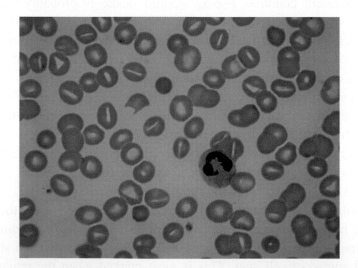

Fig. 4.6. PB film from a patient taking excess alcohol showing anaemia, marked macrocytosis and numerous stomatocytes. Note that, in contrast to megaloblastic anaemia, the neutrophil is normally segmented.

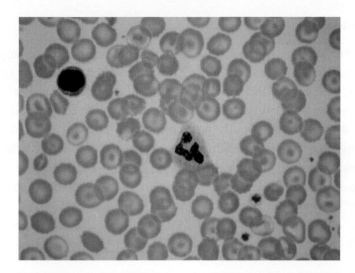

Fig. 4.7. PB film from a patient with obstructive jaundice showing macrocytosis and target cells.

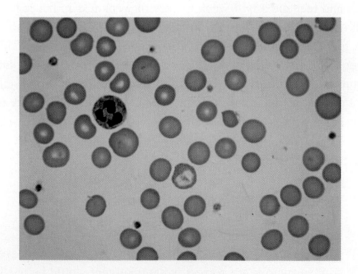

Fig 4.8. PB film from a patient with glucose-6-phosphate dehydrogenase deficiency and acute haemolysis showing macrocytosis as a result of marked reticulocytosis. It is clear that the polychromatic cells are larger than other erythrocytes.

Conclusion

The correct diagnosis in patients with macrocytic anaemia is important since missing a deficiency state can lead to a patient becoming severely pancytopenic and, in the case of vitamin B_{12} deficiency, can permit the progression of neurological damage that may not be reversible. The correct diagnosis can usually be made on the basis of clinical history including drug history, vitamin B_{12} and folate assays, and liver and thyroid function tests. If the diagnosis is still not clear a bone marrow aspirate is indicated. If the diagnosis still proves difficult, a trial of vitamin B_{12} and folic acid therapy is indicated. Assays of methylmalonic acid and homocysteine can also be useful in diagnostically difficult cases.

Test Case 4.1

A 55-year-old Caucasian school teacher presents to her general practitioner with a four-month history of numbness and tingling in her hands and feet and a two-week history of weakness in her legs. She is on no medications, has a normal diet, takes 1–2 units of alcohol each night and does not smoke. On examination, she has reduced power and brisk tendon reflexes in her legs, an extensor plantar response, reduced proprioception and vibration sense to the ankles and a normal appreciation of light, touch and heat. Laboratory tests show normal liver and renal function, Hb 11 g/dl (normal range [NR] 11.8–14.8) and MCV 103 fl (NR 82–98). The WBC and platelet count are normal.

Questions

1. What is the most likely diagnosis and why?
2. What other tests would you do next and what would you expect?
3. If your suspicions are correct, what treatment would be needed?

Write down your answers before checking the correct answer (page 323) or re-reading any relevant parts of the chapter.

5

Haemoglobinopathies and Haemolytic Anaemias

What Do You Have to Know?

☞ The structure and function of the red cell membrane (outline only)

☞ The role of the glycolytic pathway and the pentose shunt in maintaining the integrity of the red cell

☞ The inheritance, clinicopathological features, diagnosis and management of sickle cell anaemia

☞ That there are other forms of sickle cell disease

☞ The clinicopathological effects of other significant haemoglobinopathies (outline only)

☞ How haemolysis and haemolytic anaemia are defined

☞ The mechanisms and causes of haemolytic anaemia

☞ How haemolytic anaemia is diagnosed

☞ The clinicopathological effects, diagnosis and management of representative hereditary and acquired haemolytic anaemias — hereditary spherocytosis, hereditary elliptocytosis, pyruvate kinase deficiency, glucose-6-phosphate dehydrogenase deficiency, autoimmune haemolytic anaemia and haemolytic–uraemic syndrome

☞ The function of the spleen and the consequences of hyposplenism

Introduction

An erythrocyte passes through the heart half a million times and travels 300 miles in its 120-day life span. It is subject to deformation as it squeezes through capillaries only a third of its own diameter. As well as physical trauma, the red cell is exposed to endogenous and exogenous oxidants that can oxidise both membrane and intracellular constituents including haemoglobin. It is particularly vulnerable to damage as it passes from splenic cords to splenic sinuses. To survive the vicissitudes of its life, the red cell needs to generate energy, protect itself against oxidant damage, maintain its haemoglobin in the reduced form, enhance oxygen delivery from haemoglobin and maintain a flexible semipermeable membrane. In addition to the capabilities of mature red cells, reticulocytes can synthesise proteins; they are thus able to synthesise haemoglobin whereas mature red cells have no ribosomes and have thus lost the capacity for protein synthesis.

The disciform erythrocyte has 40% more membrane than a sphere of the same size. This is very important for its flexibility. It is also important that the concentration of haemoglobin is not abnormally high within the red cell or there is an increase in internal viscosity, again reducing deformability.

The red cell membrane

The red cell membrane is a lipid bilayer with integral membrane proteins supported by a cytoskeleton composed of spectrin, actin and other proteins (Fig. 5.1). It serves to maintain the shape and flexibility of the red cell and to pump ions and water across the membrane.

The glycolytic pathway

The erythrocyte derives energy from glycolysis, also known as the Embden–Meyerhoff pathway (Fig. 5.2). Energy is necessary for the ion pumps which maintain an ion gradient across the red cell membrane and prevent swelling or shrinking of the cell. In addition, the glycolytic pathway leads to synthesis of 2,3 disphosphoglycerate (2,3 DPG), also know as 2,3 biphosphoglycerate (2,3 BPG), which enhances oxygen delivery

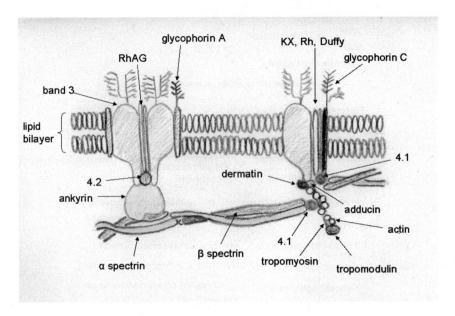

Fig. 5.1. Diagram of the red cell membrane and cytoskeleton. The red cell membrane is composed of a lipid bilayer composed of similar amounts of cholesterol and phospholipids; cholesterol is disposed equally between the two layers whereas phospholipids are asymmetrically disposed. Phosphatidyl choline and sphingomyelin are mainly in the outer leaflet while phosphatidylethanolamine and phosphatidyl serine are mainly in the inner leaflet. There are more than 100 integral membrane proteins; some having a transport function and some connecting the lipid bilayer to the underlying cytoskeleton. The cytoskeleton is composed of dimers of α and β spectrin which are assembled into a network of tetramers. The transmembrane band 3 and RhAG proteins bind to protein 4.2 and ankyrin; ankyrin binds to spectrin. The lipid bilayer is also tethered to the cytoskeleton by glycophorin C, KX, Rh and Duffy, which bind to protein 4.1 and thus to spectrin. Band 3 also binds to adducin and dermatin. In addition to these vertical interactions, spectrin binds to protein 4.1 and thus to actin microfilaments, creating horizontal interactions. It is these highly complex interactions that maintain the shape and the flexibility of the red cell.

from a haemoglobin molecule that has already given up one oxygen; it does this by binding with greater affinity to deoxyhaemoglobin and allosterically favouring the release of further oxygen molecules. 2,3 DPG thus contributes to co-operativity (see page 2). Increased synthesis of 2,3 DPG in circumstances of increased need helps the body to adapt to anaemia, living at high altitude and chronic hypoxia due to disease.

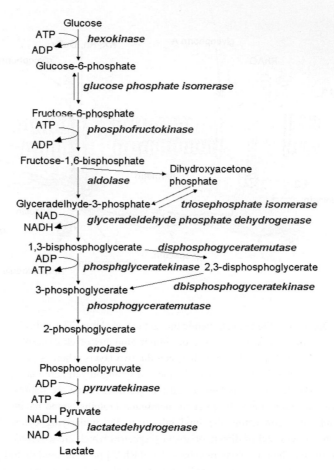

Fig. 5.2. Diagram of the glycolytic pathway. Enzymes are shown in red and metabolites in black. Glycolysis provides adenosine triphosphate (ATP), needed for red cell ion pumps. Some adenosine triphosphate (ATP) is converted to adenosine diphosphate (ADP) in the early steps of glycolysis but overall there is net production of ATP. NAD = nicotinamide–adenine dinucleotide.

The pentose shunt

The pentose shunt, also known as the hexose monophosphate shunt, is very important in the erythrocyte since it generates nicotinamide-adenine dinucleotide phosphate (NADPH) and reduced glutathione and thus protects the cell from oxidant damage (Fig. 5.3). It is also essential for synthesis of 5-carbon sugars and thus nucleic acids.

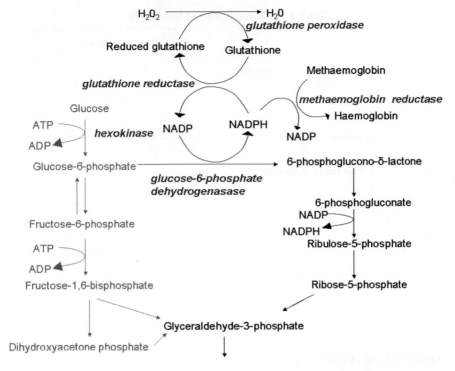

Fig. 5.3.   The pentose shunt showing how NADPH (nicotinamide–adenine dinucleotide phosphate) is generated thus permitting reduction of oxidised proteins, including methaemoglobin, and protection of the red cell from peroxides, particularly hydrogen peroxide. The glycolytic pathway is shown in grey and the pentose shunt and related pathways in black. Some key enzymes are in red.

Mechanisms of Haemolysis

Haemolysis means a shortened red cell survival. This is compensated for by an erythropoietin-driven increase in erythropoiesis. The bone marrow can increase its output of red cells five- to six-fold so there can be compensation for a red cell life span as short as 20–30 days. If the bone marrow cannot compensate, haemolytic anaemia occurs. There are inherited and acquired causes of haemolysis. Some of these are summarised, with examples, in Table 5.1. Congenital and acquired factors can interact. Thus, an inherited deficiency of glucose-6-phosphate dehydrogenase (G6PD) may only become apparent after the cell is exposed to some unusual oxidant stress.

Table 5.1. Some causes of haemolysis.

Cause	Example
Causes of congenital haemolytic anaemia	
Defect in glycolytic pathway	Pyruvate kinase deficiency
Defect in pentose shunt	Glucose-6-phosphate dehydrogenase deficiency
Defect in haemoglobin	Sickle cell anaemia, unstable haemoglobin
Causes of acquired haemolytic anaemia	
Mechanical damage	Microangiopathic haemolytic anaemia, malfunctioning prosthetic heart valve
Antibody damage	Autoimmune haemolytic anaemia
Oxidant damage	Exposure to oxidant drugs or chemicals
Enzymatic damage	Envenomation by certain snakes
Heat damage	Severe burns

Diagnosis of Haemolysis

It is possible to measure the red cell life span by labelling red cells with a radioactive isotope and thus definitively identify haemolysis. However, in practice the conclusion that there is haemolysis is made by indirect means using: (i) evidence that there is increased red cell breakdown (e.g. increased bilirubin — particularly unconjugated bilirubin — and lactate dehydrogenase [LDH], free haemoglobin in the plasma or urine, reduced serum haptoglobin, haemosiderin in the urine or increased urinary urobilinogen); (ii) evidence of increased bone marrow activity (e.g. increased reticulocyte count and the presence of polychromatic macrocytes and nucleated red cell in the blood film); (iii) abnormal red cells of a type that is found in haemolytic anaemia (e.g. spherocytes, elliptocytes, irregularly contracted cells, sickle cells, red cell fragments); or (iv) evidence for a specific type of haemolytic anaemia (e.g. a positive direct antiglobulin test or a reduced concentration of red cell G6PD). A low haptoglobin concentration provides evidence of haemolysis because, when there is intravascular haemolysis, haemoglobin released from red cells forms a complex with haptoglobin and the complex is removed by the liver. Other clinical features can also suggest haemolysis, although they are not specific for it, e.g. splenomegaly or gallstones at a young age. The gallstones in haemolytic anaemia are bile pigment stones, formed because of the increased load of bilirubin that is excreted; they may lead to acute cholecystitis and biliary obstruction.

Examples of some of the blood film abnormalities that might indicate a haemolytic anaemia are shown in Table 5.2.

The Haemoglobinopathies

The haemoglobinopathies are a group of inherited disorders in which a mutation of a globin gene leads to synthesis of a structurally abnormal haemoglobin, known as a variant haemoglobin. Such mutations can affect any globin gene but those of clinical significance mainly affect either the α or the β globin gene. The thalassaemias, which have been discussed in Chapter 3, can be regarded as a specific type of haemoglobinopathy. The possible results of a mutation in a globin gene are shown in Table 5.3. The great majority of mutations in globin genes are harmless. However, a small number of mutations that are potentially harmful are very common in certain ethnic groups, specifically haemoglobin S and haemoglobin C (in those of African ancestry) and haemoglobin E (in South-East Asia).

Sickle cell trait

Sickle cell trait or heterozygosity for haemoglobin S is not a disease. It is the carrier state for haemoglobin S. It is of genetic significance but rarely of clinical significance.

Haemoglobin S has an uncharged valine instead of a charged glutamic acid at position 6 of the β globin chain, which makes its deoxy form far less soluble than normal. The point mutation in the β globin gene that gives rise to haemoglobin S has arisen independently at least three times in different parts of Africa and also somewhere in an area extending from Arabia to India. The mutation can thus be found in people of African

Table 5.2. Some of the blood film abnormalities that might suggest haemolytic anaemia.

Abnormality	What is it and what might it mean?	Abnormality	What is it and what might it mean?
	Sickle cell: sickle cell disease		Haemoglobin C crystal: haemoglobin C disease
	Spherocyte: hereditary spherocytosis or autoimmune haemolytic anaemia		Elliptocyte: hereditary elliptocytosis
	Stomatocyte: hereditary stomatocytosis		Crenation: renal failure or pyruvate kinase deficiency (particularly post-splenectomy)
	Acanthocyte: inherited membrane defect; liver failure		Irregularly contracted cell: glucose-6-phosphate dehydrogenase deficiency or oxidant damage
	Red cell fragment (schistocyte): microangiopathic haemolytic anaemia or mechanical haemolysis		Keratocyte: oxidant damage or mechanical or microangiopathic haemolysis

ancestry and from the Indian subcontinent but is also present in a significant proportion of Arabs, Greeks and Sicilians.

Clinical features

Most individuals with sickle cell trait have no relevant clinical abnormality. Occasionally they suffer from haematuria or reduced renal concentrating ability and rarely from renal papillary necrosis. Very rarely

Table 5.3.   Types of mutation that occur in a globin gene.

The same amino acid is encoded, no phenotypic effect
A similar amino acid is encoded, no clinical effect
Haemoglobin is prone to polymerise, e.g. haemoglobin S
Haemoglobin is prone to crystallise, causing haemolysis, e.g. haemoglobin C
Haemoglobin is unstable, causing haemolysis
High-affinity haemoglobin, polycythaemia occurs
Low-affinity haemoglobin, anaemia occurs (but there is no functional effect as tissue
    delivery of oxygen is normal)
Haemoglobin is prone to oxidise, causing methaemoglobinaemia and cyanosis
Haemoglobin is synthesised at a reduced rate, e.g. haemoglobin E and the thalassaemias

an individual is exposed to hypoxia of sufficient severity to lead to signs and symptoms due to sickling. This can happen with vigorous, prolonged exercise at high altitudes, when flying in an unpressurised aircraft and if hypoxia is allowed to occur during anaesthesia.

Laboratory features

The blood count is normal. Haemoglobin electrophoresis or high-performance liquid chromatography (HPLC) shows that about 45% of the total haemoglobin is haemoglobin S, the rest being haemoglobin A and a small amount of haemoglobin A$_2$ (Fig. 5.4, lane d). The red cells can be induced to sickle in the laboratory by addition of a sample of the patient's blood to a phosphate buffer acting as a reducing agent, leading to a visible cloudiness. This is called a sickle solubility test and is necessary because not all haemoglobins that look like haemoglobin S on haemoglobin electrophoresis or HPLC are actually haemoglobin S.

Management

It is important to avoid hypoxia during anaesthesia. Testing is therefore performed before surgery in patients from ethnic groups in which this mutation is prevalent. When emergency surgery is needed, time permits only a blood count and a sickle solubility test but this should be followed by definitive testing.

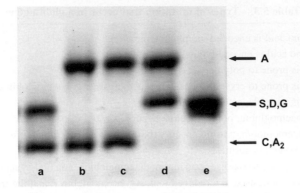

Fig. 5.4. Haemoglobin electrophoresis on a cellulose acetate membrane at an alkaline pH showing: (lane a) haemoglobin S + haemoglobin C; (lane b) haemoglobin A + haemoglobin C; (lane c) haemoglobin A + haemoglobin C; (lane d) haemoglobin A + haemoglobin S + haemoglobin A_2; (lane e) haemoglobin S + haemoglobin A_2.

The need for testing for haemoglobin S must also be considered for individuals who are planning to become pregnant or are already pregnant since there is a one in four chance of the child of two carriers of haemoglobin S having sickle cell anaemia (Fig. 5.5).

Sickle cell anaemia

Sickle cell anaemia results from homozygosity for the β^S gene and occurs when the gene is inherited from both parents. Since there are no normal β genes, haemoglobin A is totally absent (Fig. 5.4, lane e). Haemoglobin S is prone to polymerise at low oxygen tension, leading to formation of long, twisted polymers that deform the cell into the shape of a sickle. This process is reversible when the cell is again exposed to a high oxygen tension but, after several cycles of sickling, secondary changes in the cell membrane make the shape change irreversible. Sickle cell formation leads to obstruction of blood vessels and resultant tissue infarction. Vascular obstruction is due not only to the abnormal shape and the rigidity of the sickled red cell but also to secondary changes in the erythrocyte membrane, dehydration of the cell that increases internal viscosity and interaction of the sickled cell with neutrophils and endothelial cells. Intravascular haemolysis also leads

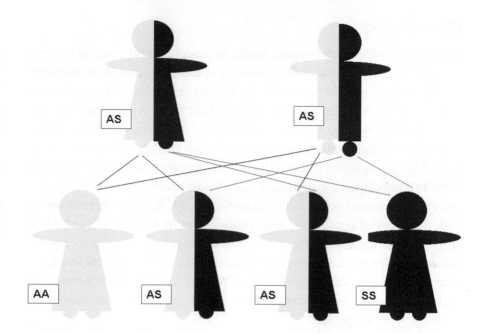

Fig. 5.5. Diagram showing the possible outcomes of a pregnancy when both parents have sickle cell trait. The β^S gene is represented in deep red and the normal β^A gene in pink. On average, a quarter of offspring will be normal, a quarter will have sickle cell anaemia and a half will have sickle cell trait.

to destruction of nitric oxide (NO), an important physiological vasodilator. Over time, recurrent infarction can lead to permanent tissue damage in multiple organs.

Red cell life span is reduced from the normal 120 days to 10–20 days so that there is hyperbilirubinaemia and an increased incidence of gall-stones. However, the low haemoglobin concentration (Hb) in sickle cell anaemia is largely because haemoglobin S is a low-affinity haemoglobin, which releases oxygen to tissues very readily. Since tissue oxygen delivery is normal, a lower Hb suffices and erythropoietic drive is less than would otherwise be expected. The hyperactivity of the bone marrow leads to an increased need for folic acid.

There are now more than 12,000 people with sickle cell disease in Britain, the majority of whom have sickle cell anaemia.

Clinical features

Patients with sickle cell anaemia suffer recurrent painful crises as a result of tissue infarction in the chest, abdomen, spine and limbs; infarction may involve bones, soft tissues or both. Pulmonary infarction can lead to hypoxia, which may be fatal. Infarction of the kidneys can cause haematuria. In children, infarction of small bones of the hands and feet can lead to painful swelling, referred to as dactylitis or the 'hand-foot syndrome' (Fig. 5.6). Young children can suffer from splenic sequestration, in which there is a rapid increase of spleen size due to pooling of red cells in the spleen and resultant severe acute anaemia; it leads to hypovolaemic shock and, if not treated rapidly and appropriately, can be fatal. In older children splenic sequestration no longer occurs because splenic fibrosis means the spleen is no longer distensible. In children, and to a lesser extent in adults, thrombosis in cerebral vessels leads to stroke. From adolescence onwards, males may suffer from priapism, as a result of obstruction of venous drainage from the penis.

Infarction due to sickling may have medium- and long-term sequelae. Recurrent splenic infarction leads to a clinically significant loss of splenic function. In considering the significance of this it is useful to think about the function of the spleen (Box 5.1). Infarction of soft tissues of the legs

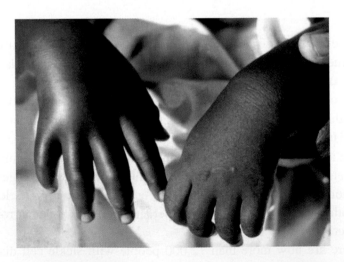

Fig. 5.6.   Dactylitis in a child with sickle cell anaemia.

can lead to chronic ulceration (Fig. 5.7). There is an increased incidence of osteomyelitis as infarcted bone is prone to secondary infection. Uncommonly, infarction of the growth plate prevents bone growth so that there is shortening of one or more fingers or toes (Fig. 5.8). Infarction of the femoral heads can lead to osteonecrosis and osteoarthritis (Fig. 5.9). Recurrent renal infarction can lead to renal failure in early middle age.

Box 5.1
The function of the spleen

Removal of senescent or damaged red cells
Antibody synthesis
Removal of encapsulated microorganisms
Removal of antibody- or complement-coated microorganisms
Removal of red cell inclusions including malaria parasites and babesia

Because of the short red cell life span, infection by parvovirus B19 (which infects red cell precursors and causes a temporary arrest in erythroblast maturation) can cause a rapid fall of Hb, leading to symptomatic anaemia.

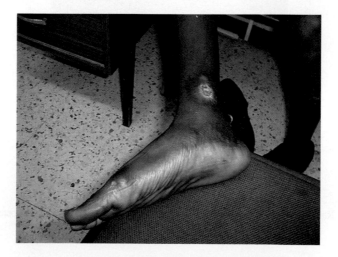

Fig. 5.7.   A leg ulcer in a patient with sickle cell anaemia.

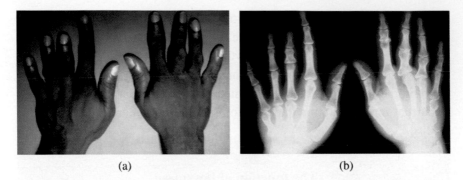

(a)   (b)

Fig. 5.8.   Clinical photograph and radiograph showing possible sequelae of bone infarction in young children with sickle cell anaemia; the third and fourth figures of the left hand are abnormally short due to shortening of the metacarpals.

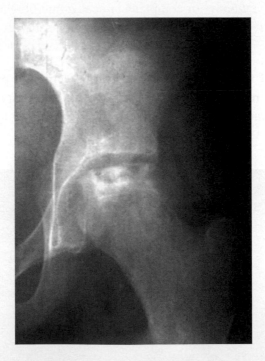

Fig. 5.9.   Radiograph showing osteoarthritis of the hip as the result of previous osteonecrosis.

Hyposplenism leads to susceptibility to blood-born infections such as those due to pneumococcus, meningococcus and *Haemophilus influenzae*. There is also susceptibility to malaria. Although sickle cell heterozygosity offers partial protection against malaria it is important to realise that sickle cell anaemia definitely does not.

Laboratory features and diagnosis

The Hb is usually around 6 to 8 g/dl with an increased reticulocyte count. The blood film shows sickle cells, target cells, polychromasia, nucleated red blood cells and the features of hyposplenism (Howell–Jolly bodies, Pappenheimer bodies and an increased platelet count; Fig. 5.10). A sudden fall of the Hb to lower levels can be the result of splenic sequestration, folic acid deficiency leading to megaloblastic anaemia or infection by parvovirus B19. Parvovirus causes a temporary arrest of erythropoiesis which passes unnoticed in people with a normal red cell life span but in patients with a shortened red cell life span can cause symptomatic worsening of the anaemia; a very low reticulocyte count is a clue to this complication.

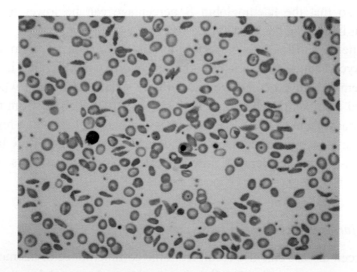

Fig. 5.10. Blood film of a patient with sickle cell anaemia showing numerous sickle cells, target cells, one lymphocyte and one nucleated red cell. There are some Howell–Jolly bodies and large platelets as an effect of hyposplenism.

Haemoglobin electrophoresis or HPLC shows haemoglobins S, A_2 and F with a total absence of haemoglobin A.

Biochemical tests show an increased bilirubin (particularly unconjugated) and LDH, both as a result of haemolysis.

Management

Children with sickle cell anaemia require vaccination against pneumococcus, meningococcus and *Haemophilus influenzae*. They should also be prescribed prophylactic penicillin which ideally should continue for life. Prophylactic folic acid is also advised. Parents should be instructed as to how to palpate the abdomen to recognise the enlarged spleen of splenic sequestration and seek urgent medical advice if this is suspected.

During a sickle cell crisis the patient needs adequate analgesia and avoidance of dehydration, hypoxia and cold. If there is infection, antibiotics are required. Splenic sequestration requires urgent transfusion and parvovirus infection can also necessitate transfusion. However, transfusion should not be used to treat the chronic anaemia of sickle cell anaemia. Patients with hypoxia due to a severe chest crisis require exchange transfusion so that the haemoglobin S percentage can be lowered rapidly without increasing the blood viscosity.

Patients suffering from recurrent crises can benefit from regular hydroxycarbamide (previously known as hydroxyurea), which increases the haemoglobin F percentage and reduces sickling. Children who have suffered a stroke, or who are at high risk of stroke, benefit from regular blood transfusion to lower the percentage of haemoglobin S. A high risk of stroke is recognised by Doppler measurements of blood flow in cerebral vessels, an accelerated flow indicating that the vessel is already narrowed.

Other forms of sickle cell disease

Sickle cell disease can also result from the co-inheritance of haemoglobin S from one parent and either β thalassaemia or a haemoglobin that interacts with haemoglobin S from the other parent. The most frequent are sickle cell/β thalassaemia and sickle cell/haemoglobin C disease. In sickle cell/β thalassaemia there may be a small amount of haemoglobin A (if the thalassaemia gene is a β^+ gene) or absent haemoglobin A (if the thalassaemia gene is a β^0 gene). In either instance there is microcytosis. In sickle cell/haemoglobin C disease there are equal amounts of haemoglobin S and haemoglobin C (Fig. 5.4 lane a); haemoglobin C does not have a reduced oxygen affinity so the Hb is higher than in sickle cell anaemia, even being normal in some patients.

Red Cell Membrane Defects

Defect in the cytoskeleton that supports the red cell membrane can cause haemolytic anaemia. Inherited abnormalities that can lead to haemolysis can occur in many of the proteins shown in Fig. 5.1, including band 3, RhAG, protein 4.2, α spectrin, β spectrin and actin. Hereditary spherocytosis and hereditary elliptocytosis will be discussed as examples of red cell membrane defects.

Hereditary spherocytosis

Hereditary spherocytosis results from an inherited defect in the red cell membrane that leads to either compensated haemolysis or a haemolytic anaemia. Estimates of frequency among Caucasians vary between 1 in 1000 and 1 in 3000. In three-quarters of instances there is autosomal dominant inheritance while in the others there is either autosomal recessive inheritance or a new mutation has occurred. Causative mutations may be in the genes encoding band 3, actin, protein 4.2, α spectrin or β spectrin. It will be seen by reference to Fig. 5.1 that these proteins are involved in vertical interactions between the red cell membrane lipid bilayer and the supporting cytoskeleton. Defects in the proteins therefore leave part of the membrane unsupported so that it is lost by vesiculation. The cell therefore becomes progressively more spherocytic as it ages, with formation of spherocytes and microspherocytes. This leads to increased rigidity so that the cell is likely to become trapped and prematurely destroyed in the spleen.

Clinical features

Patients may present with symptomatic anaemia or recurrent jaundice. There is an increased incidence of pigment gallstones. Many patients are asymptomatic.

Laboratory features and diagnosis

The blood count may or may not show anaemia. The MCHC is often increased. The reticulocyte count is increased. The blood film (Fig. 5.11) shows spherocytosis and polychromasia. Hb may be reduced or normal but the reticulocyte count is increased. Bilirubin and LDH are increased.

Diagnosis is based on the observation of a haemolytic anaemia or compensated haemolysis with spherocytosis. If there is a family history of spherocytosis no further tests are needed unless the anaemia is more severe than expected from the family history. In the absence of a family history, it is necessary to exclude the possibility of autoimmune haemolytic anaemia, an alternative cause of spherocytosis, by demonstrating a negative direct antiglobulin test. The diagnosis of hereditary

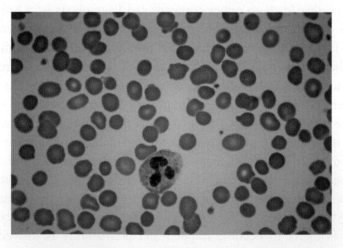

Fig. 5.11. Blood film of a patient with hereditary spherocytosis showing a neutrophil and numerous spherocytes — small dark cells that lack central pallor.

spherocytosis can be confirmed by showing reduced binding of a dye, eosin-5-maleamide, to red cells (detected by measuring fluorescence on flow cytometry). An osmotic fragility test is also abnormal but this test is now rarely performed.

Management

The anaemia responds to splenectomy but if anaemia is mild it is better to avoid the risks of splenectomy. There is an increased need for folic acid so this is often prescribed. Some patients require surgery for gallstones. It should be noted that if splenectomy is required patients must be protected, as far as possible, from the adverse effects of hyposplenism (Box 5.2).

Box 5.2
Protection from post-splenectomy sepsis

Vaccination against pneumococcus (appropriate vaccine for age), meningococcus C and *Haemophilus influenzae* type B (performed at least two weeks before splenectomy when possible)

Lifelong prophylactic oral penicillin (or erythromycin if allergic to penicillin)

When travelling: avoid malaria, be aware of the risk of babesia, have quadrivalent meningococcal vaccine before travel to certain countries

Seek urgent treatment for dog bites (because of the risk of serious *Capnocytophaga canimorsus* infection)

Carry a card or wear an alert bracelet or pendant advising of hyposplenic state

---

Hereditary elliptocytosis

Hereditary elliptocytosis usually causes only mild compensated haemolysis but occasional patients have haemolytic anaemia. Its prevalence is highest in West Africa, where it occurs in around 2% of individuals, but it is not infrequent among Caucasians. Inheritance is autosomal dominant.

Hereditary elliptocytosis can result from mutation in genes encoding protein 4.2, α spectrin and β spectrin. Reference to Fig. 5.1 shows that these
proteins are concerned with horizontal interactions and the stability of the
cytoskeleton. Mutations lead to mechanical instability and erythrocytes
become elliptocytic with a reduced surface to volume ratio as they age.

Clinical features

Most individuals with hereditary elliptocytosis are asymptomatic and the
diagnosis is an incidental one. Occasionally there is symptomatic anaemia.

Laboratory features and diagnosis

Diagnosis is based on the distinctive blood film (Fig. 5.12), usually with
compensated haemolysis but sometimes with haemolytic anaemia.

Management

Usually no treatment is necessary but rarely, when haemolysis is severe,
splenectomy is required.

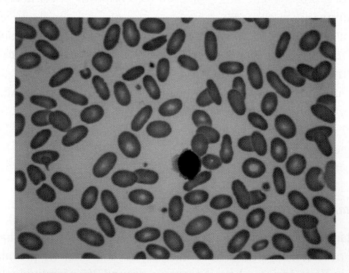

Fig. 5.12.   Blood film of a patient with hereditary elliptocytosis showing a lymphocyte
and numerous elliptocytes.

Defects in the Glycolytic Pathway

An intact glycolytic pathway leads to a net gain in adenosine triphosphate (ATP), which meet the energy needs of the red cell (Fig. 5.2). Defects in this pathway therefore lead to shortened red cell survival. All defects of the glycolytic pathway are rare.

Pyruvate kinase deficiency

Pyruvate kinase deficiency is the most common of the rare defects in the glycolytic pathway. Although deficiency is infrequent, it occurs in many ethnic groups. The blood count, reticulocyte count and biochemical tests indicate a chronic haemolytic anaemia. The blood film shows no specific abnormality. Diagnosis is by assay of enzyme activity. When haemolysis is severe, splenectomy may be needed.

Defects in the Pentose Shunt

Deficiency of G6PD is common in many populations worldwide. Other defects in the pentose shunt are rare. The pentose shunt maintains oxygen in its normal functional reduced form. When the pentose shunt is defective and the red cell is exposed to oxidant stress, haemoglobin is oxidised to the non-functional methaemoglobin, which is incapable of oxygen transport.

Glucose-6-phosphate dehydrogenase deficiency

The gene encoding G6PD is on the X chromosome so that most affected individuals are male. However, symptomatic deficiency can also occur in homozygous females and, occasionally, in heterozygous females. G6PD deficiency is common in populations from around the Mediterranean (Italians, Greeks, Cypriots, Arabs) and also in Afro-Caribbeans and others of African ancestry. In the great majority of cases, presentation is with neonatal jaundice or with acute intermittent haemolysis. Rarely, when deficiency is severe, there is chronic haemolysis.

Clinical features

Most individuals with G6PD deficiency are asymptomatic until oxidant stress to the red cells leads to acute haemolysis. Such oxidant stress may be reactive oxygen species generated by neutrophils during an infection or may be attributable to ingestion of broad beans or a drug (such as primaquine or dapsone) or exposure to a chemical (such as naphthalene). The previously well individual develops haemoglobinuria, jaundice and acute anaemia.

Babies with G6PD deficiency have an increased incidence of neonatal jaundice, not necessarily accompanied by anaemia since it is in part due to the effect of G6PD deficiency on hepatic cells.

Laboratory features and diagnosis

The blood film confirms the anaemia and shows irregularly contracted cells (Fig. 5.13). Sometimes the haemoglobin is precipitated in half of the cell, leaving the rest of the red cell membrane empty, a 'hemighost,' and sometime the red cell has lost all its haemoglobin during intravascular lysis and has become an empty membrane, a 'ghost cell' (Fig. 5.13). A Heinz body preparation is positive, indicating that methaemoglobin is present (Fig. 5.14). There is rapid development of polychromasia and the reticulocyte count rises.

The blood film is very important in diagnosis. A G6PD assay confirms the diagnosis but sometimes results are normal during acute haemolysis because of the high reticulocyte count (reticulocytes have a higher concentration of the enzyme). It is then necessary to repeat the assay after the acute haemolytic episode is over.

Management

Following acute haemolysis, the anaemia may be severe enough to require transfusion. Otherwise, prevention is important. The patient must be given an accurate list of drugs that can cause haemolysis and doctors caring for such patients should check a reliable list (e.g. the British National Formulary) before prescribing.

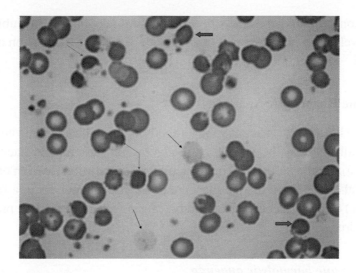

Fig. 5.13. Blood film of a patient with acute haemolysis as the result of exposure to an oxidant drug in a patient with G6PD deficiency. There are irregularly contracted cells (red arrows), ghost cells (black arrows) and hemi-ghost cells (blue arrows). The haemolysis is very recent so that, although the anaemia is severe, there is not yet any polychromasia.

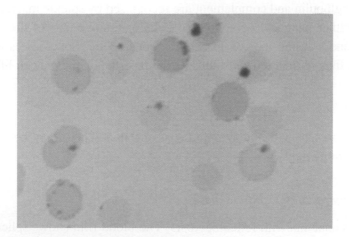

Fig. 5.14. A Heinz body preparation in a patient with G6PD deficiency and acute haemolysis showing numerous Heinz bodies (brilliant cresyl blue stain). The erythrocytes have stained pale blue; the Heinz bodies are the large deep blue inclusions within the erythrocytes.

Neonatal jaundice should be managed by keeping the bilirubin at a safe level, using phototherapy. Occasionally, exchange transfusion may be needed.

Immune Haemolytic Anaemias

Immune haemolytic anaemia is an antibody-mediated haemolytic anaemia. The antibody may be an autoantibody (as in autoimmune haemolytic anaemia), an alloantibody (as in a haemolytic transfusion reaction or when maternal antibodies cross the placenta and cause haemolysis in a fetus or neonate) or a drug-dependant antibody (causing haemolysis in the presence of the drug).

Autoimmune haemolytic anaemia

Autoimmune haemolytic anaemia results from development of an antibody directed at autologous erythrocyte antigens. This can occur as part of a recognised autoimmune disease, such as systemic lupus erythematosus, or the autoimmune process may be confined to the red cells. Erythrocytes are coated by immunoglobulin, with or without complement components. Immunoglobulin and complement are recognised by splenic macrophages, which either phagocytose entire red cells or remove part of the red cell membrane, causing the cell to become spherocytic. Spherocytes are less flexible than normal red cells, thus further shortening the red cell life span.

Clinical features

Patients present with the symptoms of anaemia. There may be jaundice and splenomegaly.

Laboratory features and diagnosis

There is anaemia with reticulocytosis. The blood film shows spherocytes and polychromasia. Biochemical evidence of haemolysis is present. The diagnosis is confirmed by a positive direct antiglobulin test (also known as a Coombs' test). This is a test for the identification of immunoglobulin and complement on the red cell membrane.

Management

Treatment is initially with corticosteroids. If the disease is not easily controlled, other immunosuppressive agents may be added. In severe cases, splenectomy may be needed.

Microangiopathic Haemolytic Anaemia

This is a type of haemolytic anaemia resulting from a pathological process in small blood vessels that causes fragmentation of red cells. The capillaries may have abnormal endothelial cells and contain fibrin strands that trap and damage red cells. There are many causes including haemolytic uraemic syndrome, thrombotic thrombocytopenic purpura (see Chapter 11) and metastatic tumour. The blood film detection of red cell fragments is important in making the diagnosis.

Haemolytic–uraemic syndrome

This syndrome typically occurs in young children and usually results from infection by a specific strain of *Escherichiae coli*, *E. coli* O157:H7. This pathogenic *E. coli* secretes verocytotoxin, which damages endothelial cells, particularly in the kidney, leading both to fragmentation of adherent red cells and to renal failure. There is diarrhoea followed by the onset of jaundice and clinical features of anaemia. Laboratory tests show anaemia, reticulocytosis, red cell fragments, increased bilirubin and LDH, and increased creatinine. The haemolysis is reversible once the acute phase of the illness is over. If appropriately managed, if necessary by haemodialysis, the renal failure is also reversible in most cases.

Conclusions

Haemolytic anaemia can be suspected when there is evidence of increased breakdown of red cells, increased bone marrow response and red cells of abnormal appearance. The diagnosis depends on an initial blood count and blood film with further specific tests being indicated by the blood film abnormalities. Sickle cell anaemia has many clinicopathological manifestations of which haemolytic anaemia is one; other features are related directly or indirectly to vascular obstruction and tissue infarction. Other haemolytic anaemias are also one feature of a serious systemic disease, such as haemolytic–uraemic syndrome or autoimmune haemolytic anaemia secondary to systemic lupus erythematosus.

Test Case 5.1

A 25-year-old woman presents with right upper quadrant pain, nausea and vomiting. On examination, she has tenderness in the right upper quadrant and scleral icterus. Ultrasonography of the abdomen shows a number of gallstones in the gall bladder. On specific questioning she admits that occasionally in the past she has noticed yellowness of her eyes. A blood count shows: WBC $13 \times 10^9/l$, neutrophil count $10.8 \times 10^9/l$, Hb 10 g/dl (normal range [NR] 11.8–14.8), MCV 101 fl (NR 82–98) and platelet count $407 \times 10^9/l$. A blood film shows spherocytes and polychromatic macrocytes, so further tests are done. The reticulocyte count is $250 \times 10^9/l$ and the direct antiglobulin test is negative. Bilirubin is increased and is mainly unconjugated.

Questions

1. Are you surprised that a 25-year-old has gallstones?
2. What is the most likely diagnosis and why?
3. Why was a direct antiglobulin test done and what does it tell us?

Write down your answers before checking the correct answer (page 324) or re-reading any relevant parts of the chapter.

Test Case 5.2

A 5-year-old Afro-Caribbean girl has been known to have sickle cell anaemia since birth, when the diagnosis was made after neonatal screening. She had an episode of dactylitis at the age of 18 months and suffers from painful crises several times a year. She takes penicillin and folic acid regularly. Her mother brings her to the Paediatric Accident and Emergency Department because she appears very listless and is thought to be paler than normal. On examination, there is no jaundice and the spleen is not felt. A blood count shows: WBC 9.6×10^9/l, Hb 3.5 g/dl (normal range [NR] for a 5-year old girl 10.0–14.0), MCV 87 fl (NR 75–90) and platelet count 313×10^9/l. A blood film shows sickle cells, target cells and Howell–Jolly bodies but polychromasia is noted to be absent. A reticulocyte count is 2×10^9/l (NR 50–100 $\times 10^9$/l).

Questions

1. What does the reticulocyte count tell us?
2. What is the most likely diagnosis and why?
3. How should the child be managed?

Write down your answers before checking the correct answer (page 324) or re-reading any relevant parts of the chapter.

6

Miscellaneous Anaemias, Pancytopenia and the Myelodysplastic Syndromes

What Do You Have to Know?

☞ The causes, diagnosis and management of normocytic normo-chromic anaemias (including renal failure and aplastic anaemia)
☞ The possible causes of pancytopenia and how they are recognised
☞ The nature, diagnosis and management of aplastic anaemia
☞ The nature, clinicopathological features, diagnosis and principles of management of the myelodysplastic syndromes

Normocytic Normochromic Anaemia and Other Miscellaneous Anaemias

Some of the causes of normocytic normochromic anaemia and associated diagnostic features are shown in Table 6.1. The clinical history and physical examination are of considerable importance in making a specific diagnosis. If no specific diagnosis is suggested from the history and examination, it can be useful to examine a blood film and measure serum ferritin, serum vitamin B_{12}, red cell folate, serum creatinine and the erythrocyte sedimentation rate as an initial step.

Table 6.1.   Some causes of normocytic normochromic anaemia.

Causative conditions	Diagnostic features
Early iron deficiency*	Low serum ferritin
Early anaemia of chronic disease*	Increased rouleaux and erythrocyte sedimentation rate, low serum iron, normal or high serum ferritin
Double deficiency of iron and vitamin B_{12} or folic acid	Hypersegmented neutrophils, low ferritin and either low serum vitamin B_{12} or low red cell folate
Blood loss	If blood loss is severe and acute, anaemia is leucoerythroblastic; polychromasia and reticulocytosis develop within a few days
Some haemolytic anaemias[†]	Polychromasia, increased reticulocyte count, increased serum bilirubin and lactate dehydrogenase, possibly specific poikilocytes
Some myelodysplastic syndromes[†]	Other features of myelodysplastic syndromes
Renal failure	Sometimes crenation or schistocytes, creatinine elevated
Liver failure[†]	Target cells, stomatocytes, acanthocytes, other cytopenias, abnormal liver function tests
Multiple myeloma[†]	Increased rouleaux and erythrocyte sedimentation rate when serum paraprotein is present
Hypothyroidism[†]	Low thyroxine and high thyroid stimulating hormone
Addison's disease and hypopituitarism	Lymphocytosis, eosinophilia, neutropenia, monocytopenia
Anorexia nervosa	Small numbers of acanthocytes, sometimes other cytopenias
Pure red cell aplasia[†]	Reticulocyte count very low or reticulocytes absent; may have a thymoma, lymphoproliferative disorder or autoimmune disease

* Can also be microcytic.
[†] Can also be macrocytic.

Renal disease

Renal disease may be complicated by microangiopathic haemolytic anaemia, which is a feature of severe hypertension, the haemolytic–uraemic syndrome (see page 101) and thrombotic thrombocytopenic purpura (see below). Renal failure has haematological manifestations, causing both anaemia and impaired platelet function. Renal failure may result from haematological diseases, such as sickle cell disease and multiple myeloma. All adults who present with renal failure should be tested urgently for myeloma as renal damage may be initially reversible.

Renal failure

Anaemia in renal failure is multifactorial. An important mechanism is inadequate erythropoietin synthesis but there may also be shortening of red cell survival. In acute renal failure there may be a more pronounced haemolytic element. When renal failure results from multiple myeloma, bone marrow infiltration contributes to the anaemia.

The anaemia of chronic renal failure may benefit from recombinant erythropoietin therapy. For maximum effectiveness, iron stores must be adequate so that maintaining the serum ferritin above100 $\mu g/l$ is recommended. The aim of therapy should be a haemoglobin concentration of 10–11 g/dl since higher levels are not associated with a better quality of life or other outcome and may have adverse cardiovascular effects. A rapid rise of haemoglobin concentration (Hb) should also be avoided, since this may cause hypertension.

Thrombotic thrombocytopenic purpura

This is a rare condition characterised by some or all of a pentad of clinical features: fever, neurological abnormalities, renal impairment, microangiopathic haemolytic anaemia and thrombocytopenia. It is caused by an autoantibody to Von Willebrand factor-cleaving protease (ADAMTS13). Deficiency of this protease leads to an excess of ultralarge multimers of von Willebrand factor, which causes a thrombotic microangiopathy with platelet consumption. Although this condition is rare, its rapid recognition is important because there is a high mortality in the absence of specific treatment. Detection of a low platelet count and red cell fragmentation is an appropriate clinical setting is important in the initial recognition of the condition. It is not necessary to have all features of the pentad to make a provisional diagnosis. Treatment is by plasma exchange, possibly supplemented by immunosuppression. Platelet transfusions should not be used since their use may aggravate the tissue ischaemia.

Liver disease

Anaemia in liver disease may be normocytic normochromic or macrocytic and may be accompanied by other cytopenias. Haematological abnormalities are multifactorial. The effects of excess alcohol consumption and folic acid deficiency may be superimposed on those of liver disease and patients with cirrhosis may develop portal hypertension leading to hypersplenism with associated pancytopenia. The blood film may show macrocytes, stomatocytes (Fig. 6.1) or target cells. There are two specific types of haemolytic anaemia associated with liver disease. Zieve's syndrome refers to acute haemolysis and hyperlipidaemia associated with alcoholic fatty liver (Fig. 6.2). Spur cell haemolytic anaemia refers to haemolytic anaemia associated with a severe acanthocytic change, occurring in liver failure of any aetiology (Fig. 6.3).

Pancytopenia

Pancytopenia refers to a reduction in the total white cell count (WBC), neutrophil count, Hb and platelet count. There are many possible causes,

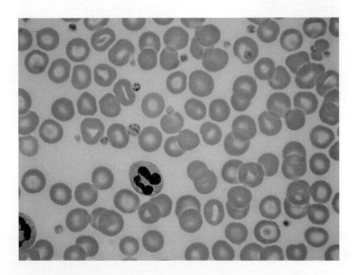

Fig. 6.1. Peripheral blood (PB) film showing macrocytes, stomatocytes and target cells in a patient with portal cirrhosis.

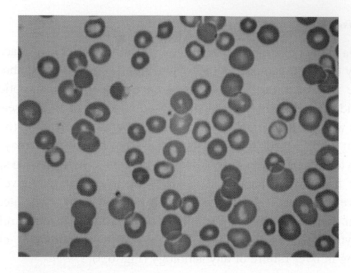

Fig. 6.2. PB film showing several irregularly contracted cells and some polychromatic macrocytes in a patient with Zieve's syndrome.

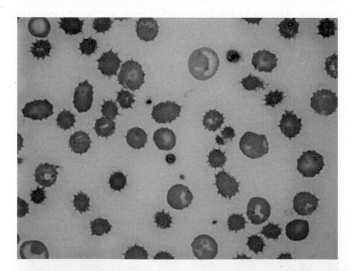

Fig. 6.3. PB film showing polychromatic macrocytes and a severe acanthocytic change in a patient with terminal liver failure and spur cell haemolytic anaemia.

which will often be apparent from the clinical history or suggested by blood film features (Table 6.2).

In current medical practice pancytopenia is often the effect of administration of anti-cancer or immunosuppressive drugs and is an expected side effect of the treatment. Much less often it results from radiotherapy.

Patients with acute leukaemia usually present with a high WBC but sometimes with pancytopenia. Particularly in children, pancytopenia may be the result of infiltration of the bone marrow by the lymphoblasts of acute lymphoblastic leukaemia. There may be clinical features such as

Table 6.2. Some causes of pancytopenia.

Cause	Possible diagnostic clues
Bone marrow suppression by drugs (e.g. anti-cancer drugs or immunosuppressive agents) or irradiation	Clinical history
Severe megaloblastic anaemia (including the effects of methotrexate therapy)	Macrocytes, hypersegmented neutrophils
Bone marrow replacement by leukaemic blast cells	Clinical features (splenomegaly ± lymphadenopathy), some blast cells in peripheral blood
Bone marrow infiltration by metastatic carcinoma	Clinical features, leucoerythroblastic blood film with teardrop poikilocytes
Primary myelofibrosis	Splenomegaly (which is often marked), leucoerythroblastic blood film with teardrop poikilocytes
Myelodysplastic syndromes	Red cell anisocytosis and poikilocytosis or a dimorphic population, dysplastic changes in neutrophils, large or hypogranular platelets,
Aplastic anaemia	None
Human immunodeficiency virus (HIV) infection	Clinical history, opportunistic infections, lymphopenia
Osteopetrosis	Leucoerythroblastic blood film
Hypersplenism	Clinical or blood film features of liver disease, splenomegaly

splenomegaly and lymphadenopathy and the blood film usually shows at least a small number of lymphoblasts. Replacement of the normal marrow by myeloid blast cells can similarly cause pancytopenia in patients of any age with acute myeloid leukaemia (AML). The blood film is likely to show at least some blast cells or other abnormal myeloid cells.

Pancytopenia can result from replacement of the bone marrow by non-haematological cells, e.g. metastatic carcinoma cells. There is often associated fibrosis, which contributes to the cytopenia. The patient may have a history of previous cancer or may have systemic features such as weight loss. The blood film often shows the presence of nucleated red blood cells and myelocytes, this being known as a leucoerythroblastic anaemia.

Pancytopenia can result from a marked reduction in the number of haemopoietic stem cells in the bone marrow (aplastic anaemia, see below) or from defective differentiation and maturation of cells derived from a defective stem cell (myelodysplastic syndromes, see below).

Pancytopenia can occur despite normal bone marrow function if the spleen is very large and blood cells are being pooled in the spleen. This is a feature of portal hypertension in patients with cirrhosis. It also occurs in Gaucher's disease when the spleen contains many Gaucher's cells; in this condition partial replacement of the bone marrow by Gaucher's cells also contributes to the pancytopenia. In primary myelofibrosis (see page 194), pancytopenia is due both to hypersplenism and to progressive fibrosis of the bone marrow.

Aplastic anaemia

Despite its name, aplastic anaemia is characterised by pancytopenia rather than just anaemia. The reticulocyte count is low and the blood film shows no specific morphological abnormality. Bone marrow biopsy shows that haemopoietic marrow is replaced by fat cells (Fig. 6.4). Aplastic anaemia may be due to an inherited genetic abnormality (Fanconi anaemia and dyskeratosis congenita). It can be due to drug exposure, either to excessive doses of a drug that regularly causes bone marrow suppression (such as a cytotoxic agent) or to normal doses of a drug to which the patient suffers an idiosyncratic reaction. Drugs that can cause permanent bone marrow damage as an idiosyncratic reaction include chloramphenicol, phenylbutazone,

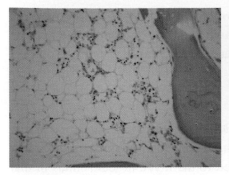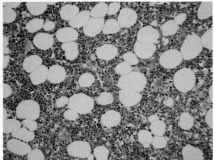

Fig. 6.4. Trephine biopsy section from a patient with aplastic anaemia (left) showing that most of the bone marrow cavity between the bones is occupied by fat cells. In comparison, a normal marrow (right) shows active haemopoiesis with the fat cells being a much smaller proportion of the intertrabecular space.

phenytoin, chlorpropamide and tolbutamide. The Epstein–Barr virus can lead to aplastic anaemia but mainly in individuals with a defective immune response to the virus. Some cases of aplastic anaemia occur a few months after an attack of what appears to be hepatitis; however, there is no proof that this hepatitis results from viral infection and an underlying autoimmune process has been postulated. Some cases of aplastic anaemia are idiopathic (i.e. no cause is discovered).

Treatment available includes immunosuppressive treatment and allogeneic stem cell transplantation. Immunosuppressive treatment is usually anti-lymphocyte globulin (produced by immunising horses or rabbits) plus ciclosporin. The basis of its success is that in many cases of aplastic anaemia there is damage to haemopoietic cells by suppressor T lymphocytes. In patients with less severe aplastic anaemia, anabolic steroids may be of benefit. Acute myeloid leukaemia sometimes develops in patients with aplastic anaemia who have responded to immunosuppressive treatment.

Pure red cell aplasia

Aplasia may affect only the erythroid lineage. The earliest morphologically recognisable red cell precursors, proerythroblasts, are present but maturing cells are markedly reduced or virtually absent. Known causes include infection by parvovirus B19 and an autoimmune process, the latter sometimes associated with thymoma. Parvovirus-induced pure red cell aplasia is transient in people with normal immunity but may be clinically manifest in patients with haemolytic anaemia.

The Myelodysplastic Syndromes

The myelodysplastic syndromes (MDS) are a heterogeneous group of disorders that are characterised by a cellular bone marrow but, paradoxically, peripheral cytopenia. They are related to the myeloid leukaemias in that normal bone marrow cells are replaced by a clonal population of cells derived from a single mutated haemopoietic stem cell. The progeny of this stem cell retain the ability to proliferate but their maturation is abnormal in two ways. First, there is an increased rate of death of haemopoietic precursors in the marrow; this is known as ineffective haemopoiesis and is the explanation of the combination of a hypercellular marrow and peripheral cytopenia. Second, the maturation appears abnormal when cells are viewed down the microscope; this is referred to as 'dysplasia', hence the term myelodysplastic syndrome. Cells may also be functionally abnormal. In addition to ineffective and dysplastic haemopoiesis, there is a third characteristic of the abnormal clone of cells. They are genetically unstable. As a result of further mutation, a sub-clone of more malignant cells may emerge, leading to disease progression and transformation to AML.

Among the dysplastic features most typical of these syndromes are hypogranularity and hypolobulation of neutrophils (Figs. 6.5 and 6.6) and the presence in the bone marrow of either small or hypolobulated megakaryocytes (Figs. 6.7 and 6.8). Among red cell changes, one of the most characteristic is macrocytosis (Fig. 6.9). Bone marrow erythroblasts may show abnormalities such as bi- or multi-nuclearity, nuclear lobulation, nuclear fragmentation and megaloblastosis. Sideroblastic erythropoiesis can also occur (Fig. 6.10); this means that there is a defect in haem synthesis and some of the erythroblasts in the bone marrow have a prominent ring of haemosiderin granules around the nucleus, rather than the small scattered iron-containing granules that are seen in normal erythroblasts.

In a minority of patients the bone marrow is hypocellular rather than hypercellular and such cases can be difficult to distinguish from aplastic anaemia.

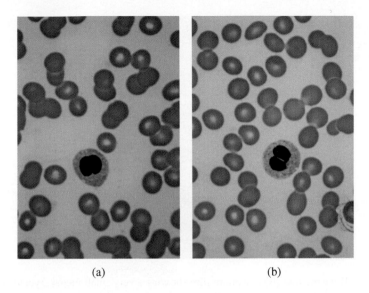

(a)   (b)

Fig. 6.5. PB film showing two hypolobulated neutrophils; the neutrophil on the right has a nucleus shaped like a pince-nez or a pair of spectacles. This is referred to as a pseudo- or acquired Pelger-Huët anomaly since the neutrophils resemble those of an inherited condition with the same name. Note that there are no platelets in the photograph so the patient clearly has severe thrombocytopenia as well.

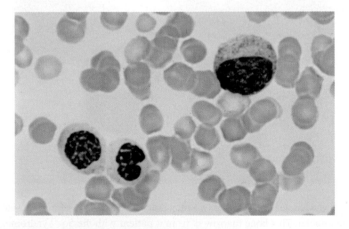

Fig. 6.6. PB film showing two neutrophils that are hypolobated and almost totally agranular. The other cell is a myelocyte. No platelets are seen.

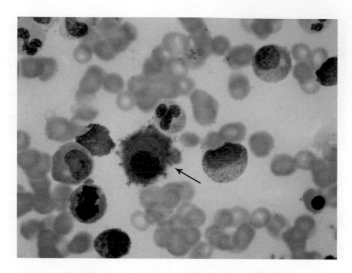

Fig. 6.7. Bone marrow (BM) aspirate film showing a very small megakaryocyte (arrow) referred to as a micromegakaryocyte.

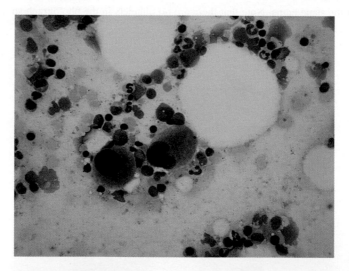

Fig. 6.8. BM aspirate film showing two megakaryocytes that are of normal size but have hypolobated nuclei. This bone marrow is from a patient with the 5q– syndrome, which is characterised by macrocytic anaemia and non-lobulated or hypolobulated megakaryocyte nuclei.

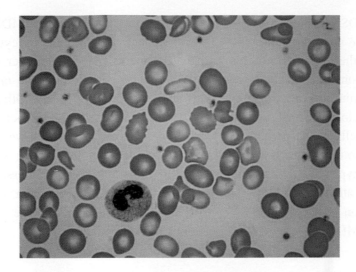

Fig. 6.9.   PB film with refractory cytopenia with multilineage dysplasia showing macro-cytosis and mild poikilocytosis. Platelet numbers appear to be normal.

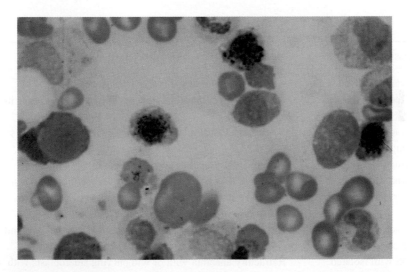

Fig. 6.10.   BM aspirate film from a patient with refractory anaemia with ring sideroblasts showing two ring sideroblasts, which have a ring of deep blue granules surrounding the nucleus. The film has been stained with a Prussian blue or Perls' stain, which stains haemosiderin.

MDS is mainly a disease of the middle-aged and elderly. MDS may arise *de novo* but some cases follow damage to stem cells by cytotoxic chemotherapy or irradiation and these patients may be younger. These conditions vary in their severity. Some cause chronic anaemia or other cytopenia but are compatible with survival for many years. Others are much closer to AML with cytopenia being combined with an increase of blast cells in the peripheral blood, bone marrow or both; however, the increase in blast cells is less than that in acute myeloid leukaemia. Some of the types of MDS are summarised in Table 6.3. MDS progresses over time. Patients with MDS can die of complications of cytopenia, such as infection or haemorrhage, or death can occur when the disease evolves into AML. This type of AML responds poorly to treatment.

Clinical features

Common clinical features result from anaemia and include fatigue, breathlessness and ankle swelling. Patients with a low neutrophil count or

Table 6.3.   **Some of the types of myelodysplastic syndrome.**

Classification	Characteristics
Refractory anaemia	Anaemia without any increase in blast cells
Refractory cytopenia	Neutropenia or thrombocytopenia without any increase in blast cells
Refractory anaemia with ring sideroblasts	Sideroblastic anaemia without any increase in blast cells
Refractory cytopenia with multilineage dysplasia	Anaemia or cytopenia with dysplasia in more than one lineage (in comparison with dysplasia confined to a single lineage in the three categories above) but without any increase in blast cells
Refractory anaemia with excess of blasts	Anaemia and dysplasia with increased blast cells in blood or bone marrow
MDS with isolated del(5)(q)	Refractory anaemia with or without ring sideroblasts with no increase in blasts cells and with isolated 5q- shown on cytogenetic analysis
Therapy-related MDS	MDS following cytotoxic chemotherapy or irradiation, often has multilineage dysplasia and may have an increase of blast cells

with a normal count but defective neutrophil function may be susceptible to infection. Patients with thrombocytopenia or defective platelet function are subject to bruising and bleeding.

On physical examination there may be pallor, bruising, petechiae and sometimes splenomegaly.

Laboratory features and diagnosis

The blood film usually shows either a normocytic or macrocytic anaemia with a variable degree of anisocytosis and poikilocytosis. In sideroblastic anaemia there is usually a major population of macrocytes and a minor population of hypochromic microcytes (Fig. 6.11); some cells contain Pappenheimer bodies, small navy blue inclusions that represent haemosiderin (Fig. 6.12). In addition to hyposegmented and hypogranular neutrophils, there may be some blast cells (Fig. 6.13). Platelets are often reduced in number and they may have reduced granules or be larger than normal.

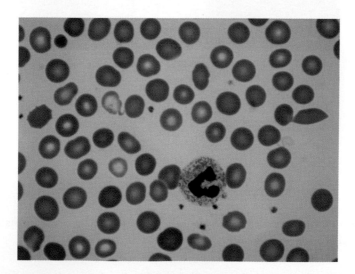

Fig. 6.11. PB film from a patient with refractory anaemia with ring sideroblasts showing a major red cell population of well haemoglobinised macrocytes and a minor population (two cells) of hypochromic microcytes. This is referred to as a dimorphic blood film.

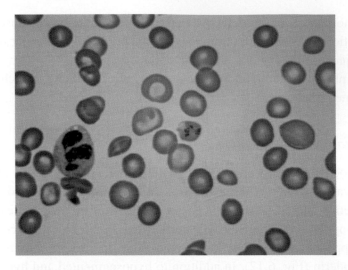

Fig. 6.12.   PB film from a patient with refractory anaemia with excess of blasts (who had sideroblastic erythropoiesis) showing a red cell (centre) containing Pappenheimer bodies.

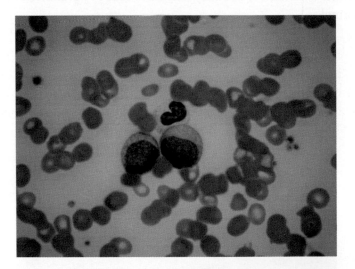

Fig. 6.13.   PB film from a patient with refractory anaemia with excess of blasts showing two blast cells and a hypogranular neutrophil band form.

The bone marrow is hypercellular with dysplastic changes in one or more lineages and sometimes an increase of blast cells. Iron stores are often increased and ring sideroblasts may be present.

Cytogenetic analysis may show an acquired clonal chromosomal abnormality, which helps to confirm the diagnosis. In the type of MDS designated MDS with isolated del(5)(q), also known as the 5q– syndrome, the clonal abnormality is an interstitial deletion of part of the long arm of chromosome 5. Other cytogenetic abnormalities can also be present including three copies of chromosome 8 (trisomy 8), loss of one copy of chromosome 7 (monosomy 7) or loss of part of the long arm of chromosome 7.

Management

Management may be symptomatic (palliative) or directed at prolonging life. Occasionally, in younger fitter patients, treatment may be directed at cure.

Symptomatic management includes use of blood transfusion or erythropoietin injections for anaemia. Erythropoietin may be more efficacious in combination with granulocyte colony-stimulating factor. Platelet infusions are used, when needed, for bleeding. Infections require antibiotics. Active management, directed at life prolongation, is with cytotoxic chemotherapy. As this is a disease particularly of the elderly, active treatment is not always indicated. Patients with the 5q– syndrome are particularly responsive to lenalidomide and azacytidine is of benefit in patients with monosomy 7. Immunosuppressive treatment can be of use, particularly in patients with a hypocellular bone marrow. In younger fitter patients, bone marrow transplantation should be considered since it offers the possibility of cure.

In patients with an otherwise good prognosis who are dependent on blood transfusions, tissue damage from iron overload can become a problem. This can be managed by chelation therapy.

Conclusions

The cause of anaemia or pancytopenia is often suggested by the clinical history and physical examination. In other circumstances, the blood film suggests a diagnosis. When the likely cause is not at all apparent, extensive investigation may be needed including haematological and biochemical tests, a bone marrow aspirate and trephine biopsy and imaging investigations.

Test Case 6.1

A 56-year-old woman presents with a lump in her breast and is found to have a carcinoma of the breast with metastasis to axillary lymph nodes. She is treated with surgery, radiotherapy and cytotoxic chemotherapy and makes a good recovery. However, seven years later, during routine follow up, she complains of fatigue and ankle swelling. Other than pallor, no abnormality is found on physical examination so some blood tests are done. A full blood count shows: WBC $3.5 \times 10^9/l$, neutrophil count $1.0 \times 10^9/l$, Hb 9 g/dl (normal range [NR] 11.8–14.8), MCV 105 fl (NR 82–98) and platelet count $96 \times 10^9/l$. The blood film is reported as showing hypogranular 'Pelger' neutrophils, a dimorphic red cell population (normochromic macrocytic cells and hypochromic microcytic cells) with Pappenheimer bodies in some erythrocytes and occasional blast cells. Liver and renal function, calcium and phosphate are all normal.

Questions

1. What is your differential diagnosis and what is the most likely diagnosis?
2. Is her past medical history relevant?
3. What should be done next?

Write down your answers before checking the correct answer (page 325) and re-reading any relevant part of the chapter.

7

Leukocytosis, Leucopenia and Reactive Changes in White Cells

What Do You Have to Know?

☞ The causes of a high white cell count and of increased numbers of neutrophils, lymphocytes and eosinophils
☞ The causes of a low white cell count, neutropenia and lymphopenia
☞ The reactive changes that occur in the blood in infection and inflammation

Leucocytosis

Leucocytosis means an increase in the white blood cell count (WBC). It is most often due to an increase in either neutrophils or lymphocytes but occasionally the number of eosinophils is sufficiently increased to cause an increase in the WBC. It is not useful to think about the causes of leucocytosis. Rather one must think about the causes of an increased number of cells of a specific cell type. It is the absolute number of cells that must be assessed rather than the percentage. For each cell type it is necessary to relate the patient's count to a normal range, when necessary a range for a specific age, gender or ethnic group.

Neutrophilia

Neutrophilia means an increase in the absolute number of circulating neutrophils. The normal range is higher in neonates than at other times of life; it is higher during pregnancy and even higher during labour and in the early post-partum period. The normal range is somewhat higher in women than in men. Neutrophil counts in people of African ancestry are often lower than in those of other ethnic origins.

Neutrophilia can be a physiological response to vigorous exercise, neutrophils that are marginated against the endothelium of blood vessels being mobilised into the circulating neutrophil pool. The same thing can happen in an epileptic convulsion or following injection of adrenaline (epinephrine). Neutrophilia is also a common, non-specific response to infection (particularly bacterial infection), inflammation (including gout and acute inflammation in connective tissue disorders) and tissue damage or necrosis (infarction, trauma, surgery, burns). The neutrophil count is increased by corticosteroid administration, as a response to blood loss or haemolysis and as a rebound phenomenon following previously low levels.

When there is neutrophilia as a response to infection or tissue inflammation or damage, there are often accompanying morphological changes such as toxic granulation, Döhle bodies and vacuolation (Fig. 7.1). 'Toxic granulation' is not specifically related to any toxin, but refers to heavy granulation as a reactive change. Döhle bodies are small oval blue-grey cytoplasmic inclusions that contain aggregates of ribosomes; they indicate cytoplasmic immaturity. These reactive changes may be accompanied by a left shift; this term indicates that the proportion of non-lobulated neutrophils (neutrophil band forms) is increased and that there are neutrophil precursors in the circulation. The presence of neutrophil vacuolation correlates strongly with bacterial infection but otherwise these reactive changes are not specific for infection. Occasionally, however, phagocytosed bacteria are seen within neutrophils, permitting rapid confirmation of the diagnosis of infection (Fig. 7.2).

Uncommonly, neutrophilia occurs as a feature of a haematological neoplasm, the neutrophils being part of the leukaemic clone of cells. This can occur in chronic myeloid leukaemia and in the myeloproliferative neoplasms (see Chapters 8 and 9). In these cases reactive changes are absent.

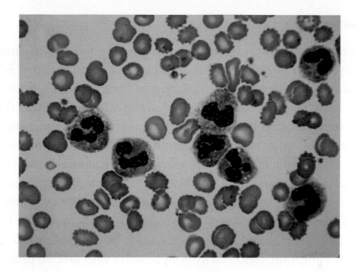

Fig. 7.1. Peripheral blood (PB) film from a patient with a bacterial infection showing neutrophilia, toxic granulation and mild neutrophil vacuolation. Two of the cells are band forms and there is therefore also a left shift.

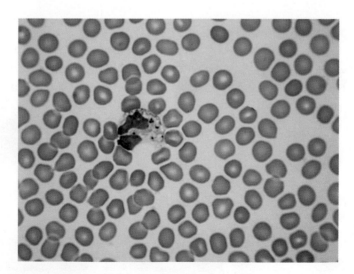

Fig. 7.2. PB film from a patient with meningococcal septicaemia showing a neutrophil that has phagocytosed meningococci. Note that there are no platelets in the film. There is severe thrombocytopenia as a result of platelet consumption through disseminated intravascular coagulation.

Lymphocytosis

Lymphocytosis means an increase in the absolute number of circulating lymphocytes. The lymphocyte count is higher in children than in adults but there are no gender or ethnic differences. Lymphocytosis is a common response to viral infection. It is also typical of whooping cough (Fig 7.3) and is sometimes seen in other bacterial infections including brucellosis and tuberculosis, and also in toxoplasmosis (infection by a protozoan parasite). Children often respond to infections, even bacterial infections, with a lymphocytosis. Acute stress, for example myocardial infarction, trauma or sickle cell crisis, can cause a sharp rise in the lymphocyte count; this is of brief duration and is followed by lymphopenia. There may be lymphocytosis early in the course of illness related to human immunodeficiency virus (HIV) infection, followed by lymphopenia with disease progression. The lymphocyte count is also increased after removal of the spleen. Allergic reactions to drugs can cause lymphocytosis.

During a lymphocyte response to viral infection there are sometimes striking changes in the cytological features of the lymphocytes. These

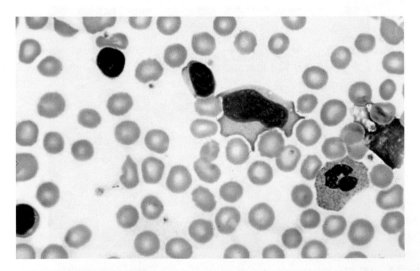

Fig. 7.3. PB film from a child with pertussis (whooping cough) showing lymphocytosis. Most of the lymphocytes are mature small lymphocytes but there is one large atypical lymphocyte with a deeply basophilic cytoplasmic margin. The photograph also shows a neutrophil and a smear cell.

reactive lymphocytes are often referred to as 'atypical lymphocytes' or 'atypical mononuclear cells'. They are increased in size with basophilic cytoplasm, cytoplasmic margins that appear to flow around adjoining red cells and a large nucleus that may have a prominent nucleolus. Atypical lymphocytes are particularly characteristic of primary infection by the Epstein–Barr virus (EBV) but they also occur in other viral infections (cytomegalovirus, hepatitis A, adenovirus, primary HIV infection), rickettsial infections, toxoplasmosis and hypersensitivity reactions to drugs.

In children and young adults, lymphocytosis is almost always reactive. In older adults lymphocytosis may be the result of a lymphoid neoplasm, either chronic lymphocytic leukaemia or non-Hodgkin lymphoma (see Chapter 8). The lymphocytes then have characteristic cytological features, which differ from those seen in reactive conditions.

Infectious mononucleosis

Infectious mononucleosis or 'glandular fever' is an illness resulting from primary EBV infection. It usually occurs in adolescents and young adults. Clinical features include fever, pharyngitis, tonsillar enlargement, lymphadenopathy and sometimes splenomegaly, jaundice or a rash. A diagnostically important laboratory feature is lymphocytosis with there being numerous atypical lymphocytes (Fig. 7.4). A minority of patients are anaemic as a result of production of an autoantibody directed at the i red cell antigen; this antibody is an agglutinating antibody acting at low temperatures so that red cell agglutinates are seen in blood films. Some patients have thrombocytopenia.

Diagnosis is usually suspected from the blood film features in an appropriate clinical context. It can be confirmed by demonstration of a specific type of heterophile antibody, a heterophile antibody being one directed at an antigen of another species. In this case the antibody agglutinates sheep or horse red cells, is absorbed by ox red cells and is not absorbed by guinea pig kidney. Simple laboratory tests are available that show these rather curious serological specificities. The diagnosis can also be confirmed by demonstrating immunoglobulin (Ig) M antibodies to EBV viral capsid antigen.

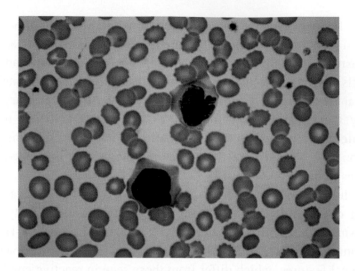

Fig. 7.4. PB film from a patient with infectious mononucleosis showing two atypical lymphocytes. These cells are enlarged in size, have large irregularly shaped nuclei and have plentiful basophilic cytoplasm that appears to be flowing around adjacent red cells. The irregular shape of the red cells (crenation) is due to delay in making the blood film.

Eosinophilia

Eosinophilia means an increase in the absolute number of eosinophils in the circulation (Fig. 7.5). There is no gender or ethnic variation, higher counts previously observed in underdeveloped countries being the result of parasitic infection. A minor increase in the eosinophil count is common in individuals with allergic rhinitis (hayfever), asthma or eczema. A more marked increase may be seen not only in these atopic conditions but also in other skin conditions, parasitic infections, allergic reactions to drugs, in some connective tissue disorders (e.g. the Churg–Strauss syndrome) and as a reaction to lymphoma or other neoplasm. Much less often the eosinophils themselves belong to a clone of neoplastic cells.

The cause of eosinophilia is often readily apparent from the clinical history and physical examination. If this is not so, the possibility of a drug reaction or parasitic infection should be considered. The parasites that cause eosinophilia are nematodes (round worms) and trematodes (flukes) that invade tissues (Figs. 7.6 and 7.7). Rarely the cause is detected in a

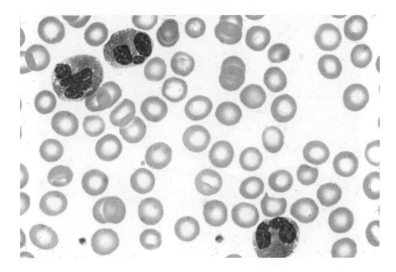

Fig. 7.5. PB film showing reactive eosinophilia. The nuclei are more lobulated than those of normal eosinophils and there are small cytoplasmic vacuoles. Minor morphological changes are common in reactive eosinophilia.

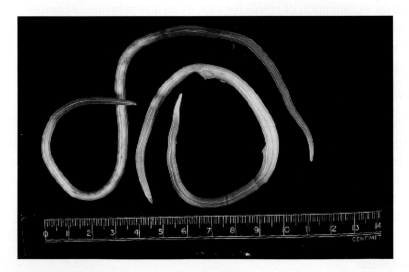

Fig. 7.6. Adult *Ascaris lumbricoides*. Eosinophilia in ascariasis is maximal during the stage of larval migration through the lungs. Reproduced with permission from Peters, W. and Pasvol, G. (2007). *Atlas of Tropical Medicine and Parasitology*, 6th Edn, Elsevier, Philadelphia.

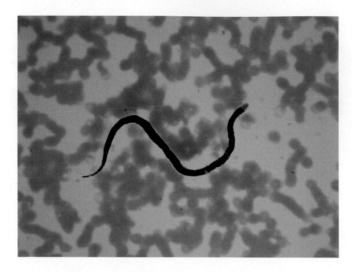

Fig. 7.7.   Microfilaria of *Loa loa* in a blood film.

blood film when microfilariae are seen (Fig. 7.7). Usually, diagnosis requires examination of stools for ova, cysts and parasites, examination of urine if schistosomiasis is a possibility and serological tests for antibodies to the more elusive parasites.

Monocytosis

Monocytosis is an increase in the number of monocytes in the circulation. It usually results from bacterial infection, including chronic infections such as tuberculosis and brucellosis. Following the more usual bacterial infections, it takes longer to appear than neutrophilia. Monocyte numbers can also be increased in inflammatory conditions, in carcinoma and as a feature of leukaemia.

Basophilia

Basophilia is an increase in the number of circulating basophils (but note that the same word also means an increased uptake of basic dyes by cytoplasm). Reactive basophilia is uncommon but basophilia is a useful diagnostic feature in myeloproliferative neoplasms and certain leukaemias, in which the basophils are part of the leukaemic clone.

Leucoerythroblastic blood response

This term means that there are nucleated red cells and neutrophil precursors in the peripheral blood film. In the neonatal period this is a normal phenomenon but at other times of life it can be diagnostically useful. It is a useful clue to the presence of bone marrow metastases or bone marrow fibrosis, including primary myelofibrosis. However, it can also occur as a physiological response to acute blood loss, haemolysis or hypoxia.

Leucopenia

Leucopenia means a decrease in the white cell count. It can be the result of a reduction in the neutrophil count, the lymphocyte count or both. As for leucocytosis, it is important to note which cell lineage is decreased.

Neutropenia

Neutropenia means a decrease in the absolute neutrophil count below the normal range, i.e. below what would be expected in a healthy individual of the same age, gender and ethnic origin. Neutropenia can be the result of a failure of bone marrow production, peripheral destruction or sequestration. Neutropenia may be multifactorial. For example, in severe bacterial infection there may be rapid migration of neutrophils to tissues with the bone marrow being unable to produce cells at a sufficient rate to maintain circulating numbers.

When neutropenia is due to a failure of neutrophil production other lineages are also often affected. Failed production can be induced by drugs or irradiation or be due to an intrinsic disorder of the bone marrow or bone marrow infiltration. Replacement of the bone marrow by abnormal cells will cause neutropenia if it is sufficiently extensive but neutropenia is most likely when there is also an intrinsic defect in haemopoietic stem cells so that differentiation to neutrophils is impaired. Neutropenia is therefore characteristic of the myelodysplastic syndromes (see Chapter 6) and acute myeloid leukaemia (see Chapter 8).

Neutrophils may be destroyed in the circulation as a result of an idiosyncratic reaction to a drug (e.g. sulphonamides or antithyroid drugs) or due to the action of an autoantibody. Neither of these is common but it is important to suspect and detect drug-induced neutropenia since continuing the drug may lead to death from overwhelming infection. Patients with severe drug-induced neutropenia, known as agranulocytosis, may have virtually no neutrophils in the peripheral blood and usually present with fever due to infection, particularly respiratory tract infection.

Sequestration of aggregated neutrophils in the lungs can occur when the circulating blood is exposed to a foreign surface, as in haemodialysis. This phenomenon is transient and has no clinical consequences.

The cause of neutropenia is often apparent from the clinical history including the drug history. The blood film may provide clues, showing dysplastic features in the myelodysplastic syndromes and acute myeloid leukaemia and a leucoerythroblastic blood film when there is bone marrow infiltration. The film often also shows reactive changes in the remaining neutrophils since secondary infection is common.

Lymphopenia

Lymphopenia or lymphocytopenia means a reduction in the absolute number of circulating lymphocytes. It is a common non-specific occurrence, being part of the body's response to stress including trauma, surgery and infection. The lymphocyte count is lowered by corticosteroids, irradiation and the administration of cytotoxic or immunosuppressive drugs. Sometimes it is of serious significance, being a feature of congenital and acquired immune deficiency syndromes.

Conclusions

An increase or decrease of a specific type of leucocyte may have an obvious cause when clinical features are considered or the blood film may offer diagnostic clues. In other patients a bone marrow examination or other tests are needed.

Test Case 7.1

A 36-year-old Somalian asylum-seeker has a health assessment, which includes blood tests and a chest radiograph. His FBC shows: WBC 3.7×10^9/l, neutrophil count 1.2×10^9/l, lymphocyte count 1.2×10^9/l, eosinophil count 1.3×10^9/l and platelet count 196×10^9/l. Hb and red cell indices (normal ranges [NR] in brackets) are:

RBC 3.71×10^{12}/l (4.32–5.66)
Hb 8 g/dl (NR 13.3–16.7)
Hct 0.26 l/l (0.39–0.50)
MCV 70 fl (NR 82–98)
MCH 21.5 (27.3–32.6)
MCHC 31 (31.6–34.9)

Questions

1. What is the likely cause of the anaemia?
2. Is there any other abnormality in the blood count that suggests an underlying cause?
3. How do you interpret the neutrophil count?

You may need to look up normal ranges for white cell counts. Write down your answers before checking the correct answer (page 325) and re-reading any relevant part of the chapter.

Test Case 7.2

A 25-year-old woman has recently been prescribed carbimazole for thyrotoxicosis. She is also taking an oral contraceptive. She presents to her GP with pharyngitis and a high fever. She looks very unwell so he does a blood count. This shows a WBC of $2.5 \times 10^9/l$ and a neutrophil count of $0.1 \times 10^9/l$. The Hb and platelet count are normal. The blood film shows marked toxic granulation. No immature cells are present.

Questions

1. What is the most likely diagnosis?
2. What action should be taken?

Write down your answers before checking the correct answer (page 325) and re-reading any relevant part of the chapter.

8

Leukaemias and Lymphomas

What Do You Have to Know?

☞ The nature of leukaemia and lymphoma and how they differ from each other
☞ For the major types of leukaemia (acute myeloid leukaemia, acute lymphoblastic leukaemia, chronic myelogenous leukaemia, chronic lymphocytic leukaemia) — the clinicopathological features, how the diagnosis is made and the principles of how the patient is managed
☞ For non-Hodgkin and Hodgkin lymphoma — the clinicopathological features, how the diagnosis is made and the principles of how the patient is managed
☞ How survival is estimated in patients with leukaemia and lymphoma
☞ When to suspect leukaemia and lymphoma and arrange urgent investigation or referral

The Nature of Leukaemia and Lymphoma

Leukaemias and lymphomas are neoplastic disorders of myeloid or lymphoid origin. They are a type of cancer. Like other cancers, they arise from a single cell that has undergone a number of mutations. These mutations give the leukaemic cells a growth or survival advantage over normal cells.

133

The leukaemic cells may proliferate more rapidly than normal cells or survive for longer. In some types of leukaemia the neoplastic cells continue
to divide but fail to mature to normal end cells.

The distinction between leukaemia and lymphoma is somewhat arbi-
trary. In general, leukaemias affect the bone marrow and often also the
peripheral blood while lymphomas develop within other tissues. However,
there is some overlap so that the same sort of cell can cause a lymphoma
in some patients and a leukaemia in others. In addition, when a lymphoma
is at an advanced stage there can be spread to the bone marrow and blood.

Leukaemias are broadly divided into lymphoid and myeloid and into
acute and chronic. Lymphoid leukaemias can be of B lineage, T lineage or
natural killer (NK) lineage. Myeloid leukaemias can affect the granulocyte
and monocyte lineages but often there is also involvement of erythroid and
megakaryocyte lineages. Which lineages are involved depends on the
type of stem cell or progenitor cell that suffered the causative mutations
(Fig. 8.1). Sometimes mutations occur in a pluripotent lymphoid myeloid

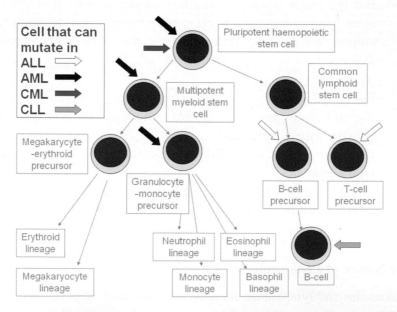

Fig. 8.1. The sites in the stem cell hierarchy where mutations can occur that give rise to
acute myeloid leukaemia (AML) or acute lymphoblastic leukaemia (ALL), chronic
myeloid leukaemia (CML) or chronic lymphocytic leukaemia (CLL).

stem cell and the leukaemic population can then include both lymphoid and myeloid cells.

The division of leukaemias into acute and chronic reflects their clinical behaviour. An acute leukaemia usually develops rapidly and, if effective treatment is not given, causes the death of the patient within a period of weeks or months. A chronic leukaemia generally has a slow onset and patients can survive many months or years, even without treatment. The clinical features result from the characteristics of the leukaemic cells. In acute leukaemia the cells are primitive cells called blast cells, either lymphoblasts or blasts of myeloid lineages (myeloblasts, monoblasts, megakaryoblasts). These cells continue to proliferate but they do not mature into normal end cells. Because of their continued proliferation without maturation, they replace the normal bone marrow cells so that bone marrow failure occurs. In chronic leukaemias maturation of leukaemic cells occurs without there being any disproportionate increase in blast cells. The end cells that are produced resemble normal mature cells.

Lymphomas are divided into Hodgkin lymphoma, also known as Hodgkin's disease, and non-Hodgkin lymphoma (NHL). Non-Hodgkin lymphoma may be of T, B or NK lineage. Initially the nature of Hodgkin lymphoma was unknown but it is now known that the neoplastic cell is of B lineage although it lacks some typical B-cell features. Non-Hodgkin lymphomas are divided into lymphoblastic lymphomas, which are very similar to acute lymphoblastic leukaemia, and lymphomas of mature T, B and NK cells. The lymphomas of mature lymphocytes are divided broadly, on the basis of their clinical behaviour, into 'high grade' and 'low grade' (or, alternatively, aggressive and indolent).

Cytogenetic and molecular changes in leukaemia and lymphoma

The mutations that give rise to leukaemia often result from changes in chromosomes that can be seen on microscopic examination. In other patients the mutation is a molecular change, occurring without any changes in chromosomes being visible. Because the leukaemic or lymphomatous cells represent a clone of cells that are the progeny of a single cell, they generally all have the same chromosomal abnormality or molecular abnormality. If a further mutation has occurred within the leukaemic clone there may be a subset of cells with a closely related rather than identical abnormality.

Chromosomal abnormalities can be detected by exposing cells in metaphase to a stain that gives each chromosome a characteristic pattern of light and dark bands. Consideration of the size and shape of the chromosomes and their banding patterns permits each pair of autosomes and the X and Y chromosomes to be identified. The abnormalities that may be detected include changes in chromosome number (loss or duplication of an entire chromosome), deletion of part of a chromosome, a translocation or an inversion. In a translocation there is movement of a chromosomal segment from one chromosome to another; usually this is an exchange of segments between two chromosomes, known as a reciprocal translocation (Fig. 8.2). In a chromosomal inversion, two breaks occur in a chromosome and the segment between the two break points flips over and joins up again the wrong way round (Fig. 8.3). An important potential result of translocations and inversions is that abnormal DNA sequences are produced. Novel genes may be produced that are composed of the 5′ end of one gene (including the promoter) and the 3′ end of another gene. These fusion genes lead to, or contribute to, the development of leukaemia or lymphoma. Often they are constitutively expressed so that cell division is uncontrolled.

Molecular changes occurring without visible cytogenetic abnormalities include point mutations, small deletions and duplications. Small deletions can alter the structure and function of a gene or, if larger, a deletion can cause the loss of a gene. Alternatively, a deletion can extend from the middle of one gene to the middle of another so that a fusion gene is produced.

Altered normal genes and new fusion genes that contribute to the development of leukaemia and lymphoma (or other cancers) are called oncogenes. The normal genes that give rise to them may be referred to as proto-oncogenes but sometimes they also are called oncogenes, because of their capacity to become oncogenic following mutation or dysregulation.

In some leukaemias and lymphomas other types of genes are also involved. These are the tumour-suppressor genes, which normally hinder

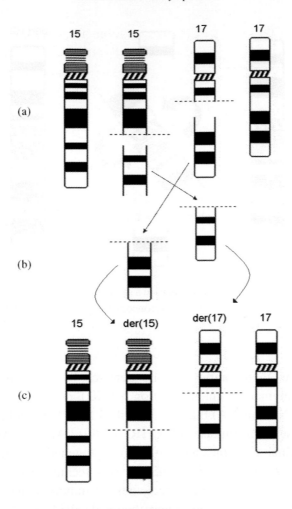

Fig. 8.2. Diagram showing how chromosomal breaking and erroneous rejoining leads to the t(15;17)(q22;q12) translocation, which is typical of acute promyelocytic leukaemia. (a) a break occurs in each chromosome; (b) crossover of the detached segments of the two chromosomes occurs; (c) the detached fragments join up to the wrong chromosome. der = derivative chromosome, i.e. a chromosome derived from a normal chromosome of the same number.

the development of leukaemias and other cancers. The inherited lack of a tumour-suppressor gene or a deletion or mutation that leads to loss of the gene or loss of its function can contribute to the development or further evolution of a leukaemia or lymphoma.

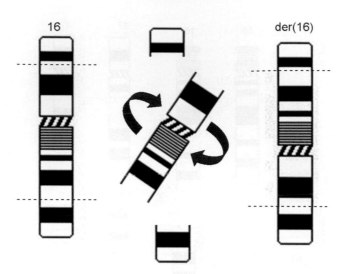

Fig. 8.3. Diagram showing how two breaks in a single chromosome, followed by inversion of the segment between the breaks and erroneous rejoining lead to inv(16)(p13.1q22), which is typical of a subtype of acute myeloid leukaemia. der = derivative chromosome.

Molecular abnormalities can be detected by DNA analysis (e.g. using the polymerase chain reaction [PCR]) or by analysis of the messenger RNA (mRNA) that is transcribed from the mutant gene (e.g. using reverse transcriptase PCR [RT-PCR]). Another very useful technique, which combines molecular and cytogenetic methods, is fluorescence *in situ* hybridisation (FISH). This technique uses probes to specific gene sequences, e.g. oncogenes or tumour-suppressor genes, which are labelled with a fluorescent chemical called a fluorochrome. By using fluorochromes that emit light of different wavelengths it is possible to combine probes for two or three genes in the one study and thus detect normal genes and fusion genes and recognise loss or duplication of genes. The chromosomes themselves can also be stained so that their size and shape can be recognised in metaphase cells (but not interphase cells). FISH is particularly useful for studying leukaemic cells that have a low mitotic rate since even if there are no cells in metaphase it is possible to count the number of signals in each cell and also recognise fusion signals.

Disease evolution

Some leukaemias and lymphomas are acute or aggressive from the beginning. In other instances further mutation occurs in one of the neoplastic cells of an initially indolent neoplastic population leading to emergence of a subclone of more malignant cells. This can lead to a chronic leukaemia transforming to an acute phase or to a low-grade lymphoma transforming to a high-grade lymphoma. Such transformations initially occur at a single site but these more malignant cells can subsequently spread widely.

Immunophenotyping

Immunophenotyping is a procedure in which expression of antigens on the surface membrane of cells but also, with modified techniques, within the cytoplasm or the nucleus, is determined. In leukaemias it is usually performed by flow cytometry using monoclonal antibodies labelled with a fluorescent chemical called a fluorochrome (Fig. 8.4). In lymphomas it is often performed on tissue section, a process called immunohistochemistry. Immunophenotyping is very important in the diagnosis of acute lymphoblastic leukaemias and chronic lymphoid leukaemias and lymphomas.

Cytochemistry

Before immunophenotyping became widely available, cytochemistry was important in determining whether an acute leukaemia was lymphoblastic or myeloblastic. Myeloblasts express myeloperoxidase (Fig. 8.5) and chloroacetate esterase and their granules also stain with Sudan black B (Fig. 8.6) while monoblasts express non-specific esterase (Fig. 8.7). Lymphoblasts give negative reactions for myeloperoxidase, Sudan black B and non-specific esterase. With the advent of immunophenotyping, cytochemical stains are much less used.

Why do people develop leukaemia and lymphoma?

There are many aetiological factors known for leukaemia and lymphoma and yet for most subtypes we do not know the cause in the majority of

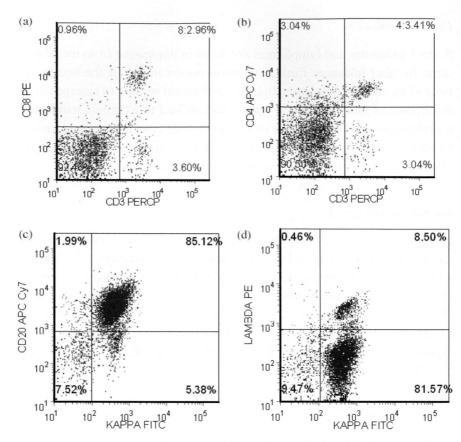

Fig. 8.4. Flow cytometric immunophenotyping used to investigate a patient with lymphocytosis and cytologically abnormal lymphocytes. In this procedure, the lymphocytes have been selected on the basis of their size and other characteristics and these results relate to cells within the lymphocyte 'gate': (a) only 6–7% of the cells are T cells (CD3 positive), some of these expressing CD8 and some not; (b) in this plot again 6–7% of the cells are T cells (CD3 positive), some expressing CD4 and some not; these two plots suggest that the bulk of the lymphocytes may be B cells; (c) 87% of the cells are confirmed to be B cells since they express CD20, a B-cell marker; the great majority of them are expressing kappa whereas normally only about two-thirds of B cells would be kappa expressing; (d) a small minority of cells are expressing lambda whereas the majority are kappa expressing, this confirming that there is a clonal population of B cells present; the small number of lambda-positive cells are residual normal B cells. FITC, PE, PERCP and APC Cy7 identify four fluorochromes that are bound to different antibodies; they emit light at different wavelengths and thus identify cells that are expressing a specific antigen. A diagnosis of non-Hodgkin lymphoma was made.

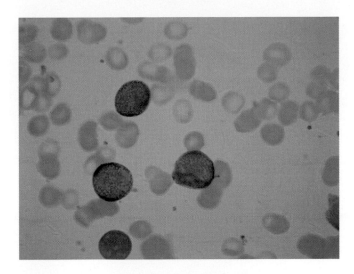

Fig. 8.5. Myeloperoxidase reaction in a patient with acute leukaemia. The reaction is strongly positive (brown) in the blast cells, thus identifying this as a case of acute myeloid leukaemia (AML).

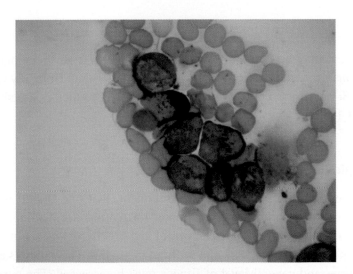

Fig. 8.6. Sudan black B staining in a patient with acute leukaemia. The reaction is strongly positive (black) in the leukaemic cells, thus identifying this as a case of AML. The particularly strong reaction is because this was a case of acute hypergranular promye-locytic leukaemia.

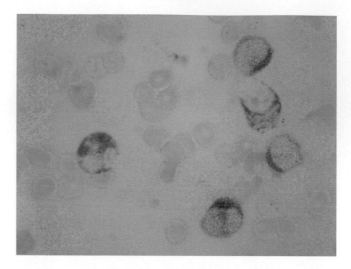

Fig. 8.7.   Mixed esterase reaction in a patient with acute leukaemia. There is positivity for both chloroacetate esterase (blue) and non-specific esterase (brown) thus indicating that in this leukaemic there is both neutrophilic and monocytic differentiation, designated acute myelomonocytic leukaemia (FAB M4 subtype).

patients. It may be that leukaemia usually results from the spontaneous mutations that occur in the human genome, rather than from any external cause. Some of the known and suspected causative factors are shown in Table 8.1.

Principles of Treatment

The general philosophy of medical treatment, that one should try to do more good than harm, is very relevant to treating haematological neoplasms. It is necessary to have a correct and precise diagnosis in order to determine the prognosis with and without treatment. The patient's age, comorbidities and general level of fitness must be assessed. The purpose of treatment in an individual patient might be: (i) relief of symptoms (palliation); (ii) prolongation of life; or (iii) cure. If the aim of treatment is to prolong life or effect a cure, decisions should be based on the best evidence available and on an assessment of the individual patient. The best

Table 8.1. Aetiological and predisposing factors for leukaemia and lymphoma.

Condition	Definite	Suspected
Acute myeloid leukaemia	Irradiation Certain immunosuppressive and anti-cancer drugs Benzene Cigarette smoking Down syndrome in infants	
Acute lymphoblastic leukaemia	Down syndrome in children (for B-lineage ALL) Irradiation *in utero*	Delayed exposure to a common pathogen (for B-lineage ALL) Certain drugs and chemicals, including *in utero* exposure
Chronic myelogenous leukaemia	Irradiation	Certain anti-cancer drugs
Chronic lymphocytic leukaemia	Familial predisposition	
B-lineage lymphomas	Epstein–Barr virus (numerous subtypes of lymphoma) Human herpesvirus 8 (several rare subtypes) *Helicobacter pylori* (one specific subtype) Immune deficiency (inherited, iatrogenic or HIV-induced) Malaria (co-factor for Burkitt lymphoma)	
T-lineage lymphomas	Human T-cell lymphotropic virus I (ATLL) Coeliac disease (EATCL)	
Hodgkin lymphoma	Familial predisposition Epstein–Barr virus Immunodeficiency (HIV)	

ATLL, adult T-cell leukaemia lymphoma; EATCL, enteropathy-associated T-cell lymphoma; HIV, human immunodeficiency virus.

evidence available will usually be derived from a randomised controlled trial or from a meta-analysis of a number of similar trials. The patient should generally be fully informed of the options available in order to make an informed decision and to give valid consent to treatment. If it is not clear that one treatment is better than another it may be appropriate to suggest entry into a clinical trial. Haematology has led the way in the use of clinical trials to determine optimal treatment for future patients.

The types of specific treatment appropriate for different haematological neoplasms include chemotherapy, molecularly targeted drug therapy, radiotherapy, immunotherapy, radioimmunotherapy and allogeneic and autologous haemopoietic stem cell transplantation (see page 282). The first question to be asked is: "Does the patient need treatment?". Some low-grade neoplasms do not need any treatment; a 'watch and wait' policy is appropriate. If treatment is needed, the second question to be asked is: "Which treatment is appropriate?". The intensity of the treatment to be given is determined by the nature of the leukaemia or lymphoma and the purpose of the treatment — palliation or life prolongation/cure. Effective treatment may have serious side effects that would not be justified if the intention was not prolongation of life or cure.

Some haematological neoplasms, e.g. myeloproliferative neoplasms, respond to non-intensive chemotherapy, often with a single oral drug. Other higher-grade neoplasms require combination chemotherapy, often incorporating parenteral as well as oral agents. The principle of combination chemotherapy is selection of drugs that are likely to be effective against the leukaemia or lymphoma but that have non-overlapping toxicities. In that way the effects on the neoplastic cells can be maximised while the toxic effects on normal tissues affect different organ systems and thus can be tolerated.

Molecularly targeted drug therapy is exemplified by tyrosine kinase inhibitors. Certain neoplasms are caused by a mutation that leads to the synthesis of an aberrant, constitutively activated, tyrosine kinase; administering a drug that is designed to inhibit this kinase may have a preferential effect on the neoplastic cells in comparison with normal cells.

Radiotherapy finds its major role in localised neoplasms, such as some lymphomas, when it is possible to administer a curative dose of radiotherapy to the tumour while sparing most normal tissues. It can also be used to treat leukaemia or lymphoma affecting the central nervous system (CNS), a site that may escape the effects of chemotherapy.

Immunotherapy includes the use of monoclonal antibodies that recognise antigens expressed on neoplastic cells; there may also be effects on normal cells expressing the same antigen. An example of such a mono-clonal antibody is rituximab; it is directed at CD20, an antigen expressed on mature B cells, and can therefore be useful in chronic lymphocytic leukaemia and B-lineage NHL. Immunotherapy can be used alone or in combination with chemotherapy. Other therapy that alters the immune response can also be of benefit since the growth of neoplastic cells is determined not only by the genetic changes in the cells themselves but also by the effect of cytokines and by the interaction of neoplastic cells with normal stromal cells. Thus, immunosuppressive therapy is of benefit is some patients with myelodysplastic syndromes (see page 112) and interferon alpha is of use in some lymphoid and myeloid neoplasms.

In radioimmunotherapy neoplastic cells are targeted by an antibody to which a radioactive isotope is bound.

Allogeneic haemopoietic stem cell transplantation ('bone marrow transplantation') may be indicated for high-grade neoplasms that cannot otherwise be cured. It is potentially efficacious for two reasons. First, it permits very high doses of chemotherapeutic agents to be given, which will kill increasing numbers of neoplastic cells. Such treatment would be likely to cause death from bone marrow failure but for the fact that the patient is 'rescued' by the donor cells. Second, the transplanted cells may include some that have a specific immune effect on the neoplastic cells, a graft-versus-leukaemia or graft-versus-lymphoma effect.

Estimating survival

There have been striking improvements in the outcome of leukaemias and lymphomas in the past two to three decades. These have resulted from improvement in supportive care and from the application of new drugs and other forms of therapy. To establish whether a proposed new form of treatment is better than what was previously available, comparisons have been made in randomised controlled trials. Such trials involve assessment of survival and also assessment of the adverse effects of treatment. Estimates of treatment-related mortality can be important when very intensive treatment is used. The meanings of some of the terms applied to clinical trials are shown in Table 8.2. Survival is usually estimated as median survival, 5-year survival or 10-year survival. Relative survival is an important

Table 8.2. Some of the ways of measuring survival in leukaemia and lymphoma trials.

Term	Meaning
Overall survival	The total length of survival, whether or not relapse has occurred
Disease-free survival	The total length of survival following treatment without relapse of the disease having occurred
Event-free survival	The total length of survival following treatment before a defined event occurs; the defined event could be relapse or a specific complication of the disease, e.g. fracture-free survival in myeloma
Progression-free survival	Survival with the disease in question not showing progression
Relative survival	Survival relative to the survival of individuals of the same age, gender and ethnic origin without the disease
Cause-specific survival	Survival without death relating to the disease in question having occurred; death from unrelated causes is excluded
Median survival	The time when half the patients are alive and half are dead (could be median overall survival, median event-free survival and so on)

measurement in population studies, being particularly relevant when a disease affects elderly persons who might die from other causes. It is important that randomised controlled trials are large enough to avoid missing a real difference in outcome between different treatment arms.

Acute Lymphoblastic Leukaemia

Acute lymphoblastic leukaemia (ALL) is predominantly a disease of childhood with a peak incidence around the age of 2–5 years. The prognosis in children is relatively good with about 85% of children being cured with modern treatment. Cases also occur in adult life with the prognosis in adults being significantly worse than in children. In adults there is a steady fall in 5-year relative survival from 45% for patients in their 20s to little over 10% in those over 60 years.

ALL is not a single disease but rather is a heterogeneous group of disorders. The majority of cases, about 75–80%, are of B lineage with the remainder being T lineage. However, a number of quite different entities are included within the B-lineage ALL category and T-lineage ALL is also heterogeneous. Many cases of ALL show an acquired clonal cytogenetic abnormality in leukaemic cells. Others show a clonal molecular abnormality. It is the nature of the cytogenetic/molecular genetic abnormalities that determines the prognosis and indicates the intensity of the treatment required. Relatively good prognosis types of B-lineage ALL include those associated with hyperdiploidy (the presence of more than the normal number of chromosomes in the leukaemic clone) and those associated with a specific acquired translocation, t(12;21)(p13;q22), in the leukaemic clone. A bad prognosis among B-lineage cases is associated with two other translocations, specifically t(4;11)(q21;q23) and t(9;22)(q34;q11.2). The t(9;22) translocation also occurs in chronic myelogenous leukaemia and in both instances is associated with a *BCR-ABL1* fusion gene. Since this translocation gives rise to an abnormal chromosome 22, referred to as the Philadelphia (Ph) chromosome, these cases are sometimes referred to as Philadelphia-positive ALL. Ph-positive ALL is uncommon in childhood but during adult life its incidence rises exponentially; this is one of the reasons why the prognosis of ALL is much worse in adults than in children. Among T-lineage cases there are also some prognostic differences that can be linked to the underlying molecular defect. Knowing the prognosis influences the treatment. Good prognosis cases are given the minimum treatment likely to be effective in order to avoid, as far as possible, the complications of treatment. Conversely, more intensive treatment, which might include stem cell transplantation, is reserved for patients in whom the prognosis is likely to be otherwise worse.

Clinical features

Clinical features can result either from the direct effects of proliferation of leukaemic cells or from bone marrow impairment as a result of crowding out of normal haemopoietic cells. Presenting features that are the direct result of tissue infiltration by leukaemic cells include bone pain, lymphadenopathy, hepatomegaly and splenomegaly. Less often there is testicular infiltration, leading to enlargement of one or both testes, or CNS infiltration, usually leading to cranial nerve palsies. Renal infiltration can

Box 8.1
Tumour lysis syndrome

Can occur in any high count leukaemia or bulky lymphoma in which
there is a high rate of cell death
Causes hyperuricaemic nephropathy and acute nephrocalcinosis
Characterised by acute renal failure with increased urea, creatinine,
uric acid, potassium and phosphate and reduced calcium

result in abdominal enlargement and impaired renal function. Patients
with a very high white cell count (WBC) can have renal failure and other
metabolic disturbance as the result of a tumour lysis syndrome (Box 8.1);
this may be present pre-treatment but is more often precipitated by
chemotherapy. In patients with T-lineage ALL, chest radiography may
show enlargement of the thymus as a result of thymic infiltration by lymphoblasts (Fig. 8.8). Presenting features resulting from impaired bone
marrow function include pallor, petechiae and bruising.

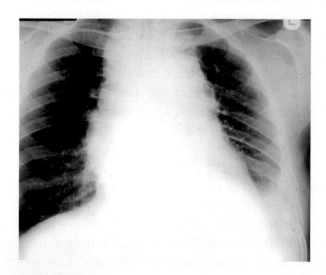

Fig. 8.8.   Chest radiograph in a patient with T-lineage acute lymphoblastic leukaemia
(ALL) showing mediastinal enlargement. There is also a small left pleural effusion.

Haematological features

There is usually anaemia and thrombocytopenia. In the majority of patients leukaemic lymphoblasts circulate in the blood (Fig. 8.9). In a minority of patients there are no circulating lymphoblasts and the diagnosis is made when a bone marrow aspirate is done to look for a cause of cytopenia.

Diagnosis and differential diagnosis

In children with cytopenia without circulating lymphoblasts the differential diagnosis includes other causes of bone marrow failure. However, if there is only isolated thrombocytopenia a diagnosis of autoimmune or post-infection thrombocytopenia is much more likely and ALL is unlikely. Once blast cells are detected in the blood or bone marrow the differential diagnosis is between ALL and acute myeloid leukaemia (AML). Since the treatment of these two types of acute leukaemia differs, immunophenotyping is essential to confirm a provisional diagnosis of ALL. Because ALL is a serious condition requiring intensive treatment it

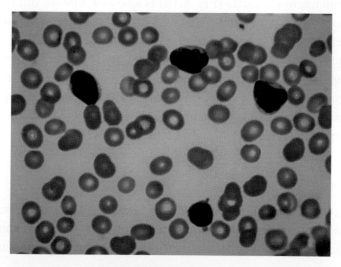

Fig. 8.9. Peripheral blood (PB) film in ALL showing three blast cells and a lymphocyte.

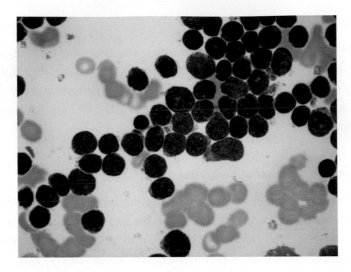

Fig. 8.10. Bone marrow aspirate film in ALL showing complete replacement of normal haemopoietic cells by leukaemic lymphoblasts.

is also necessary to do tests of liver and renal function, a uric acid assay, a coagulation screen, a blood group and antibody screen, and a chest radiograph.

A bone marrow aspirate (Fig. 8.10) is also essential for full characterisation of the disease and, because of its prognostic significance, cytogenetic analysis is always done on this aspirate. In addition, molecular analysis is always done to detect the t(12;21) translocation, which cannot usually be detected by standard cytogenetic analysis. Because of the prognostic and therapeutic importance of the t(9;22) translocation, it is necessary in adults to perform not only cytogenetic analysis but also molecular analysis for the *BCR-ABL1* fusion gene.

Management

The basis of treatment is two-fold: supportive care to compensate for the impaired bone marrow function and combination chemotherapy to attack the leukaemia. Supportive care is likely to include transfusions of red blood cells and platelets and, if the patient develops an infection, antibiotics. Careful fluid balance and prevention of hyperuricaemia is also necessary. Chemotherapy is with a combination of oral and parenteral drugs given in three phases: remission induction; consolidation; and maintenance. Maintenance treatment is continued for 2–3 years. In addition to systemic chemotherapy, it is necessary to give pre-emptive treatment to the CNS since otherwise small numbers of leukaemic cells survive in this sanctuary site and later proliferate and cause overt disease. Pre-emptive CNS therapy is usually with drugs introduced into the cerebrospinal fluid by lumbar puncture or by selection of specific drugs that can cross the blood-brain barrier. Cranial irradiation is also sometimes used. In the case of Ph-positive ALL, a tyrosine kinase inhibitor such as imatinib (see page 161) is administered in addition to combination chemotherapy. For poor prognosis ALL, allogeneic stem cell transplantation may offer the only chance of cure.

Chemotherapy has both short- and long-term toxicity. Short-term toxicity is largely reversible; it includes bone marrow suppression and other damage to normal tissues. Long-term toxicity is largely irreversible, and includes reduced fertility (especially after transplantation), mild cognitive impairment (after cranial irradiation) and a slight risk of developing AML as a result of damage to normal haemopoietic stem cells by chemotherapeutic agents. It is because of the need to balance the benefits of treatment (the chance of cure) against the risks (short- and long-term toxicity) that it is necessary to investigate patients with ALL carefully, with cytogenetic and molecular analysis, in order to determine the specific subtype of disease and the associated prognosis and thus be able to give risk-adjusted treatment.

Acute Myeloid Leukaemia

Acute myeloid leukaemia is a heterogeneous group of disorders rather than a single disease. It occurs at all ages but particularly in adults. The incidence rises ten-fold from 1 to 10/100 000 per year between the ages of 20 and 70 years. The causative mutation can occur at various levels in the stem cell hierarchy (see Fig. 8.1). Cells of the leukaemic clone continue to proliferate but show defective maturation so that there is a steady accumulation of immature cells known as blast cells in the bone marrow and usually also in the peripheral blood. These may be myeloblasts, monoblasts, erythroblasts or megakaryoblasts. Maturation may be arrested at the blast stage or there may be some residual maturation to granulocytes and monocytes. In one very specific type of AML, acute promyelocytic leukaemia, maturation to abnormal promyelocytes occurs and is arrested at that stage. Because the proliferating blast cells replace normal haemopoietic cells in the bone marrow there is a general impairment of bone marrow function. Leukaemic cells may proliferate at extramedullary sites as well as in the bone marrow. Relative survival declines markedly with increasing age and since the prevalence increases with age the overall 5-year relative survival is of the order of 20%. However, for adults between 25 and 45 years, relative survival is currently estimated at around 60%.

Clinical features

Some clinical features result directly from the proliferation of leukaemic cells; there may be splenomegaly or hepatomegaly and, less often, lymphadenopathy. Leukaemic cells can also infiltrate the skin and gums, particularly when there is monocytic differentiation (Fig. 8.11). Patients with very high white cell counts can have obstruction of small blood vessels by leukaemic cells, known as leucostasis. This can lead to stroke or respiratory impairment.

Other clinical features result from bone marrow failure. These include pallor, fatigue, dyspnoea, bruising, bleeding, petechiae and fever. Bacterial infections of the mouth and pharynx are common and can cause cervical lymphadenopathy.

Acute promyelocytic leukaemia is often complicated by disseminated intravascular coagulation (DIC) and activation of fibrinolysis so that there is prominent bleeding and bruising, for example, bruising appearing spontaneously or at venipuncture sites.

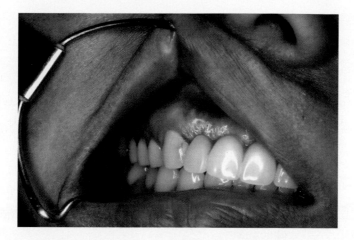

Fig. 8.11. Infiltration of the gums by leukaemic cells in acute monocytic leukaemia.

Haematological features

There is usually anaemia and thrombocytopenia. Usually the WBC is increased as a result of considerable numbers of blast cells in the peripheral blood but some patients have few or no circulating blast cells and the WBC may then be low. Blast cells may be myeloblasts, monoblasts or both. The neutrophil count is usually reduced and neutrophils can show dysplastic features. The bone marrow aspirate shows at least 20% blast cells (or in erythroleukaemia, similar numbers of very primitive erythroid cells).

AML can be classified according to whether differentiation is to myeloblasts, monoblasts, erythroblasts or megakaryoblasts. This is the basis of the French–American–British (FAB) classification (Box 8.2), first proposed 35 years ago. More recently the World Health Organisation has proposed a much more detailed and complex classification, which gives more clinically meaningful categories. The latter classification is based, as far as possible, on the cytogenetic or molecular abnormality that is responsible for the phenotypic characteristics of the leukaemia.

Box 8.2
A Summary of the FAB Classification of Acute
Smyeloid Leukaemia

M0   AML with minimal evidence of myeloid differentiation (cyto-
      chemical stains negative, immunophenotyping positive)
M1   AML without maturation
M2   AML with maturation
M3   Acute promyelocytic leukaemia
          Acute hypergranular promyelocytic leukaemia
          Acute hypogranular/microgranular promyelocytic
          leukaemia
M4   Acute myelomonocytic leukaemia
M5   Acute monoblastic/monocytic leukaemia
M6   Acute erythroleukaemia
M7   Acute megakaryoblastic leukaemia

Diagnosis and differential diagnosis

The main differential diagnoses of AML are ALL and bone marrow failure for any other reason. In many patients the diagnosis is obvious from
the clinical features plus the blood count and blood film. These patients
have blast cells with granules or rod-shaped cytoplasmic structures known
as Auer rods (Fig. 8.12) that identify the cells as blasts of myeloid lineage.
In other patients blast cells are present in the blood but cytochemistry or
immunophenotyping is needed to demonstrate that they are myeloblasts
not lymphoblasts. In some patients the diagnosis is not made until a bone
marrow aspirate is done to investigate the cause of bone marrow failure.

All patients require a bone marrow aspirate (Figs. 8.13 and 8.14);
cytogenetic analysis is performed on this aspirate to identify prognosti-
cally important subgroups (see below). When facilities exist, it is
desirable to also perform molecular analysis to identify several good
prognosis subgroups within the group of patients with normal cytogenetic analysis. Immunophenotyping is usually done in all patients and
is essential in those patients whose blasts are not obviously myeloid.

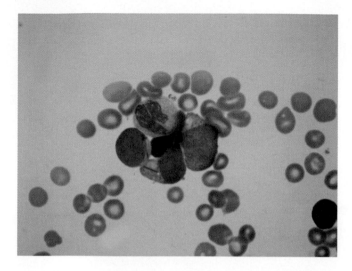

Fig. 8.12. A neutrophil and three blast cells; one of the blast cells has an Auer rod, indicating that these cells are myeloblasts.

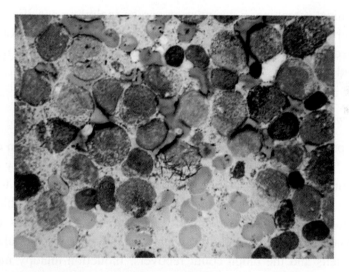

Fig. 8.13. Bone marrow aspirate in acute promyelocytic leukaemia. Most of the cells are abnormal promyelocytes with brightly staining granules. One cell in the centre contains multiple Auer rods, a characteristic feature of this subtype of AML.

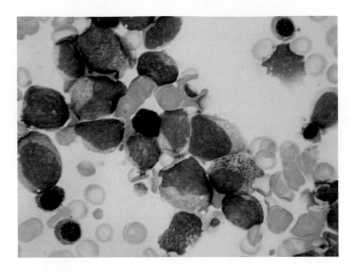

Fig. 8.14. Bone marrow aspirate in acute monoblastic leukaemia. Monoblasts are large cells with few if any granules. Their lineage can be confirmed by demonstration on non-specific esterase activity.

Biochemical screening, a coagulation screen including specific tests for DIC (particularly but not only when acute promyelocytic leukaemia is suspected), a blood group and antibody screen and a chest radiograph are indicated.

Management

Most types of AML can only be cured by intensive combination chemotherapy. This is therefore appropriate unless the patient is very elderly or has other serious illnesses that make successful treatment unlikely. The aim of initial chemotherapy, with drugs such as daunorubicin and cytarabine, is to induce a complete remission, which means that all recognisable leukaemic cells disappear, the marrow is repopulated by normal cells and the blood count recovers. Induction therapy may also include immunotherapy targeted at a myeloid antigen. Induction chemotherapy is followed by consolidation chemotherapy in an attempt to eliminate any residual leukaemic cells and prevent relapse. During this induction and consolidation therapy the patient needs support with red cell and platelet transfusions, antibiotics, antiviral therapy and, sometimes, antifungal therapy.

The optimal treatment following induction of remission depends on the subtype of leukaemia as well as on the age and general health of the patient. Cytogenetic analysis is of crucial importance in dividing AML into subtypes that differ in their prognosis and optimal treatment. For example, the presence of certain acquired cytogenetic abnormalities including the translocation, t(8;21), and the chromosomal inversion, inv(16), indicate a fairly good prognosis and the patient receives only standard combination chemotherapy; 60–70% of these patients become long-term survivors. Other chromosomal abnormalities indicate either an intermediate or a poor prognosis. The appropriate treatment may then be chemotherapy to try to induce remission followed by an allogeneic haemopoietic stem cell transplant. The potential benefits of transplantation must be weighed against the risks since transplant-related mortality is 15–30%. Some types of AML have such a poor prognosis that attempts at curative treatment are not justified. This applies to AML following previous chemotherapy in the elderly in whom only palliative care is indicated.

Acute promyelocytic leukaemia, which results from a t(15;17) translocation, is treated in a completely different way from other types of AML. Treatment is with a combination of chemotherapy and all-*trans*-retinoic acid (ATRA). Because of the specific molecular defect that results from this translocation, ATRA causes the leukaemic promyelocytes to differentiate to neutrophils, which then die. The leukaemic clone is thus almost extinguished. The chemotherapy prevents any residual leukaemic cells from subsequently proliferating and causing a relapse. This type of leukaemia is also responsive to arsenic therapy, for example with arsenic trioxide (As_2O_3). Patients with acute promyelocytic leukaemia require supportive care with fresh-frozen plasma and platelet transfusions to prevent death from haemorrhage. Diagnosis must be completed speedily and treatment instituted rapidly in order to prevent early haemorrhagic death. If this is achieved the prognosis is very good.

Chronic Myelogenous Leukaemia

Chronic myelogenous leukaemia (CML), also known as chronic myeloid leukaemia and chronic granulocytic leukaemia, is an uncommon leukaemia with the UK incidence being 1–2 per 100 000 per year. It is largely a disease of adults although childhood cases do occur. The median age of onset is 50 years and incidence increases with age. CML is more common in men than in women. This leukaemia results from a specific chromosomal translocation, designated t(9;22)(q34;q11.2), between one chromosome 9 and one chromosome 22 that leads to formation of an oncogenic fusion gene, *BCR-ABL1*, on the abnormal chromosome 22. The abnormal chromosome 22 is referred to as the Philadelphia (Ph) chromosome. Initially this is a chronic leukaemia but further mutation within a cell of the leukaemic clone leads to disease evolution to an accelerated phase and to acute transformation (Fig. 8.15). Transformation may be

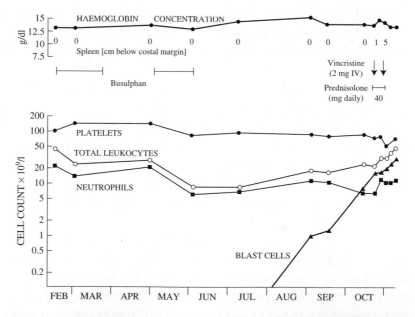

Fig. 8.15. Graphical representation of WBC and absolute counts of neutrophils and blast cells in a patient with emerging blast transformation in chronic myelogenous leukaemia. This illustration dates from a period before there was effective treatment for this type of leukaemia. Note the relentless rise of the blast cell count.

myeloid or lymphoblastic, indicating that the initial mutation that gives rise to the leukaemic clone is in a pluripotent lymphoid–myeloid stem cell. Before the availability of specific targeted treatment, this transformation was inevitable so that the median survival of patients with CML was only 2–3 years.

Clinical features

Common symptoms are fatigue, lethargy, bleeding, weight loss, splenic discomfort and increased sweating. The most common physical finding is splenomegaly; with more advanced disease the liver is also enlarged. Nowadays one-fifth or more of patients have the disease detected by an incidental blood count before the development of any symptoms.

Haematological features

There is an increase in the WBC due to an increase in both granulocyte precursors (particularly myelocytes) and in mature granulocytes — neutrophils, eosinophils and basophils (Fig. 8.16). The platelet count is usually normal or high. There may be anaemia, which is not usually

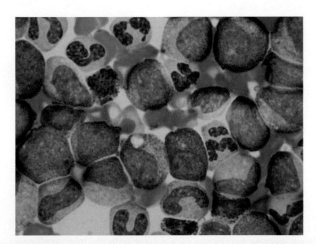

Fig. 8.16. PB film from a patient with chronic myelogenous leukaemia with a very high WBC. There are mature cells and precursors of all three granulocytic lineages.

severe. The bone marrow is intensely hypercellular due to an increase of granulocytic cells and megakaryocytes.

In the accelerated phase the peripheral blood may show thrombocytopenia or refractory thrombocytosis, basophils are often increased and there may be some increase of blast cells.

Blast crisis (particularly lymphoblastic crisis) may emerge suddenly from chronic phase disease or may follow an accelerated phase. Blast cells increase in numbers in the marrow and appear in the peripheral blood. Blast crisis may be lymphoblastic, myeloid or mixed.

Diagnosis and differential diagnosis

A marked increase in neutrophils and myelocytes, a consistent increase in basophils and usually an increase in eosinophils makes the differential count very typical so that confusion with reactive neutrophilia is only likely in early cases that are detected incidentally. Confirmation of the diagnosis requires cytogenetic analysis (Fig. 8.17)

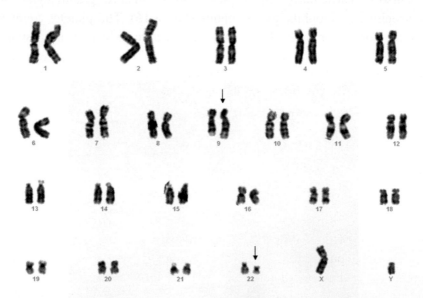

Fig. 8.17. Bone marrow karyogram of a patient with chronic myelogenous leukaemia. The two abnormal chromosomes that have been formed as a result of the t(9;22) (q34;q11.2) translocation are marked with arrows. The derivative chromosome 22 with an abbreviated long arm is the Philadelphia (Ph) chromosome.

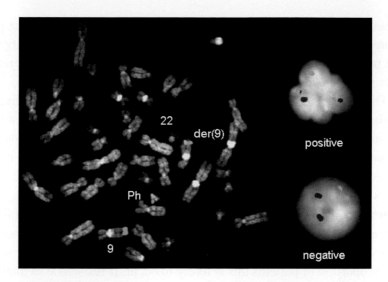

Fig. 8.18. Fluorescence *in situ* hybridization (FISH) analysis of metaphase and inter-phase bone marrow cells from a patient with chronic myelogenous leukaemia to demonstrate *BCR-ABL1* fusion. Two large differentially labelled (red and green) probes have been used, each spanning one of the chromosomal breakpoints involved in this translocation. In the presence of a translocation, each probe signal is split and two fusion signals (red–yellow–green) are seen, marking the site of *BCR-ABL1* and the reciprocal *ABL1-BCR* fusion genes. In metaphase cells (left) the fusion signals are visible on the Ph chromosome and on the abnormal chromosome 9, the derivative or der(9). This signal con-figuration is also visible in interphase cells (top right) and is easily distinguished from the pattern seen in a *BCR-ABL1*-negative cell (bottom right).

and molecular or FISH analysis (Fig. 8.18) to demonstrate the *BCR-ABL1* fusion gene.

Management

Until the end of the 1990s, CML was treated with either oral cytotoxic chemotherapy, parenteral interferon alpha or allogeneic stem cell trans-plantation. Oral chemotherapy, e.g. with hydroxycarbamide, led to a clinical and haematological remission but not to a cytogenetic remission so that acute transformation still occurred. Parenteral interferon alpha led to haematological remission and, in some patients, cytogenetic remission and, rarely, even cure. Stem cell transplantation was potentially curative but because of the possibility of death or serious morbidity from the procedure was only applicable to a subset of younger fitter patients. Targeted drug treatment has now become available, leading to a radical alteration in the management of CML.

The *BCR-ABL1* gene encodes a protein with constitutively activated tyrosine kinase function. The most effective treatment for CML is with a tyrosine kinase inhibitor, such as imatinib. In most patients this leads to a haematological remission followed by steady reduction in the size of the Ph-positive clone. In the patients with the best response, molecular techniques eventually show that *BCR-ABL1* transcripts are at a very low level or, in a small minority, are undetectable. With tyrosine kinase inhibitor treatment, the 5-year median survival is now more than 80%. It is not yet known if some patients can be cured with imatinib therapy and, if so, in what proportion of patients this is likely to occur. If resistance to imatinib develops as a result of the occurrence of a further mutation, alternative tyrosine kinase inhibitors, such as dasatinib and nilotinib, may still be efficacious. However, there are some mutations that lead to disease that is refractory to currently available tyrosine kinase inhibitors. In these refractory cases, stem cell transplantation may be indicated. In general, since the development of tyrosine kinase inhibitors, both stem cell transplantation and other forms of treatment are much less often needed.

Chronic lymphocytic leukaemia

Chronic lymphocytic leukaemia (CLL) occurs from early middle age onwards but is predominantly a disease of the elderly. The median age at presentation is in the early 70s. It is the commonest leukaemia in Western Europe and North America, with an incidence of about 3.5 per 100 000 per year. It is two to three times more common in men than in women. The disease results from proliferation of a clone of mature B cells that appear to be analogous to memory B cells.

Clinical features

In many patients the diagnosis is an incidental one and there are no symptoms or abnormal physical findings. With more advanced disease

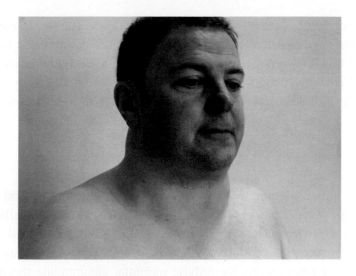

Fig. 8.19. Cervical lymphadenopathy in a patient with chronic lymphocytic leukaemia (CLL).

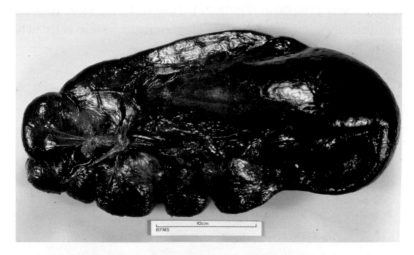

Fig. 8.20. A grossly enlarged spleen from a patient with CLL. The scale is 10 cm.

there is lymphadenopathy (Fig. 8.19), splenomegaly (Fig. 8.20), hepatomegaly and an increased susceptibility to infection. Infections are the result of low immunoglobulin concentrations and impaired cell-mediated immunity. Herpes zoster is a common occurrence. In a small number of patients there is transformation, know as Richter transformation, to a condition that resembles a large B-cell lymphoma. In some patients this does represent transformation of a CLL lymphocyte but in others it is an independent high-grade lymphoma resulting from immune deficiency and Epstein–Barr virus (EBV) infection of a non-clonal B cell.

Haematological features

There is initially lymphocytosis with an otherwise normal blood count. With more advanced disease and more extensive bone marrow infiltration there is a normocytic normochromic anaemia and thrombocytopenia. Because of the disturbed immune regulation, there is an increased incidence of autoimmune haemolytic anaemia, autoimmune thrombocytopenia and autoimmune red cell aplasia. The blood film shows a monotonous population of mature small lymphocytes with clumped chromatin and scanty cytoplasm (Fig. 8.21). These cells are more fragile than normal, leading to the formation of characteristic 'smear cells' when a

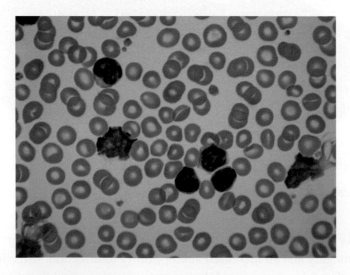

Fig. 8.21. PB film from a patient with CLL showing four small mature small lymphocytes and three smear cells.

blood film is spread. When autoimmune haemolytic anaemia occurs, there are spherocytes and polychromasia.

A bone marrow aspirate is not necessary for diagnosis if the immunophenotype is typical but, when performed, shows infiltration by similar cells to those in the blood.

Diagnosis and differential diagnosis

The differential diagnosis is with other causes of lymphocytosis, both reactive and neoplastic. Immunophenotyping is important in confirming the diagnosis since on the basis of clinical and haematological features, confusion with non-Hodgkin lymphoma can occur. Immunophenotyping shows the cells to express either kappa or lambda light chains but not both, thus providing evidence that they are monoclonal and distinguishing B-lineage neoplasms from reactive lymphocytosis, in which lymphocytes are polyclonal. The typical immunophenotype of CLL differs from that of non-Hodgkin lymphoma and provides a firm basis for the diagnosis (Table 8.3). Immunophenotyping also provides information useful in indicating prognosis. Expression of CD38 or of a protein known as ZAP70 is associated with a worse outcome. Specific cytogenetic abnormalities (detected by FISH) can also give prognostic information.

Table 8.3. Comparison of immunophenotyping in chronic lymphocytic leukaemia and B-lineage non-Hodgkin lymphoma.

	Chronic lymphocytic leukaemia[a]	Non-Hodgkin lymphoma[a]
Surface membrane immunoglobulin[b]	Weak	Moderate or strong
CD5	Positive	Negative in most subtypes
CD23	Positive	Negative
CD79b	Negative	Positive
FMC7	Negative	Positive

[a] In both conditions there will be expression of B-cell markers such as CD19, CD20 and CD22.

[b] In both conditions this is monoclonal so there is expression of either κ or λ light chain but not both.

Management

Many patients do not require treatment, this being dependent on the stage of the disease and whether there is stability or early disease progression. In patients needing treatment, this was traditionally with chlorambucil, an oral alkylating agent. The results of randomised controlled trials have shown that oral combination chemotherapy/ immunotherapy with cyclophosphamide, fludarabine and rituximab (an anti-CD20 monoclonal antibody) gives better results and this is now the treatment of choice if patients are in good general health. Chlorambucil can still be useful in frail elderly patients. Autoimmune complications usually respond well to corticosteroid therapy.

Vaccination against influenza should be given annually. Vaccination against pneumococcal infection is usually administered although antibody responses are sub-optimal. Immunoglobulin may be useful in patients with hypogammaglobulinaemia and recurrent infections. Herpes zoster should be treated promptly with an anti-viral drug, to avoid extensive disease and scarring. Patients who have received very immunosuppressive therapy, such as fludarabine, are prone to herpes virus reactivation and opportunistic bacterial and fungal infections, which require appropriate management.

Patients who have been treated with fludarabine should receive only irradiated blood products to avoid the risk of transfusion-associated - graft-versus-host disease.

Non-Hodgkin Lymphoma

Non-Hodgkin lymphoma is a neoplasm of lymphoid cells of either T, B or NK lineage. Most lymphomas are derived from cells analogous to mature lymphocytes. Those derived from lymphoblasts have many features in common with ALL and will not be discussed further. Since lymphocytes are found not only in specific lymphoid organs but also in many other tissues, NHL can arise in virtually any part of the body. At presentation, disease may be confined to a single lymph node, lymph node group or extranodal site or may be already widespread. Any lymphoma can involve lymph nodes, liver, spleen and bone marrow. Both B-lineage and

T-lineage NHL can also involve the gastrointestinal tract. Cutaneous involvement is more often due to T-lineage NHL.

There are dozens of types of NHL which differ not only in their lineage but also in their aetiology, clinicopathological features, prognosis and optimal treatment. NHL will be discussed in general terms and representative types of high-grade and low-grade NHL will then be discussed in more detail.

Clinical features

Most patients present with localised or generalised lymphadenopathy, sometimes with co-existing splenomegaly or hepatosplenomegaly (Fig. 8.22). Presentation with isolated splenomegaly also occurs. Skin infiltration may be present. When there is infiltration of the lungs or gastrointestinal tract, symptoms may relate to those organs. Waldeyer's ring, lacrimal glands, salivary glands and the thyroid are sometimes involved. Neurological symptoms occur if there is CNS involvement. There are often systemic symptoms such as malaise, fever, weight loss and sweating. Sometimes there is itch.

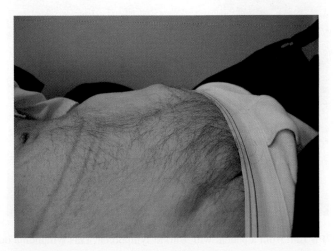

Fig. 8.22. Clinical photograph showing bilateral inguinal lymphadenopathy in a patient with non-Hodgkin lymphoma.

Haematological features

The blood count and film may be normal. In some patients there are circulating lymphoma cells (Fig. 8.23) and in others there is anaemia or other cytopenia (as a result of bone marrow infiltration) or anaemia of chronic disease (as a result of cytokine release by lymphoma cells). The erythrocyte sedimentation rate may be increased. Patients with a B-lineage lymphoma may have a paraprotein (causing increased rouleaux formation), a cryoglobulin (which may precipitate in the blood film) or a cold agglutinin (which causes red cell agglutination in the blood film).

Diagnosis and differential diagnosis

The differential diagnosis includes other causes of lymphocytosis or lymphadenopathy but since the clinical features are very variable the differential diagnosis is broad. Diagnosis is usually based either on a lymph node or other tissue biopsy supplemented by immunohistochemistry. However, diagnosis can also be based on cytology and immunophenotyping

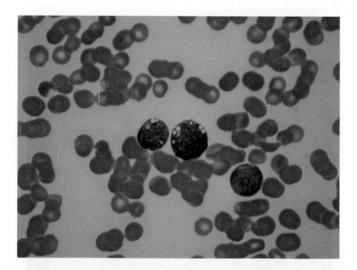

Fig. 8.23. PB film from a patient with Burkitt lymphoma. This lymphoma occurs in an endemic form in children in Africa, sporadically in developed countries and with an increased prevalence in carriers of the human immunodeficiency virus (HIV). The vacuolated strongly basophilic cytoplasm seen here is characteristic.

of circulating lymphoma cells supplemented by FISH analysis to identify the characteristic cytogenetic/molecular genetic abnormality associated with certain specific lymphomas.

Management

Management requires accurate diagnosis, an assessment of how wide-spread the disease is (known as the stage of the disease) and assessment of whether there is significant co-morbidity. Essential blood tests include tests of liver and renal function, uric acid and lactate dehydrogenase. Screening for hepatitis B, hepatitis C and the human immunodeficiency virus (HIV) is indicated in all patients since positive results will affect how the patient is managed. Lymphomas are staged as I to IV, depending on the extent of the disease, and as A or B, depending on the absence or presence of specific symptoms (fever, weight loss and night sweats; Fig. 8.24). Thus a lymphoma would be IA if it were confined to a single lymph node region and there were no symptoms whereas it would be stage IVB if there were involvement of lymph nodes, liver, spleen and bone marrow with fever and night sweats. Staging as I to IV is based on physical examination, chest radiography, computed tomography (CT) scanning of chest, abdomen and pelvis (Figs. 8.25 and 8.26) and some-times bone marrow biopsy or ^{18}F-fluorodeoxyglucose positron-emission tomography (PET scanning). Other staging investigations are performed as clinically indicated.

Treatment may be with chemotherapy, immunotherapy (monoclonal antibodies), radiotherapy or a combination of modalities. Before deciding on any specific therapy it is important to consider the aim of treatment, particularly whether or not it is realistic to aim at cure. Low-grade lymphomas can be treated with single agent oral chemotherapy but often combination chemotherapy gives better results. High-grade lymphomas require intensive combination chemotherapy supplemented, in the case of B-cell lymphomas, with rituximab. In young patients, preservation of fertility and, for men, sperm storage must be considered.

Patients who have been treated for lymphoma require long-term follow-up, both to monitor for disease progression or relapse and to detect any late adverse effects of chemotherapy or radiotherapy.

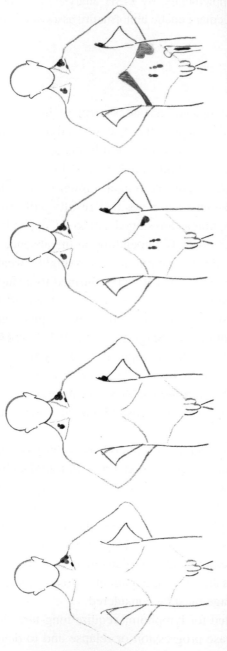

Stage I Disease confined to a single lymph node region or lymphoid structure (e.g. spleen, thymus and Waldeyer's ring)

Stage II Involvement of two or more lymphoid regions or structures but with disease confined to one side of the diaphragm

Stage III Disease on both sides of the diaphragm but with no more than limited contiguous involvement of non-lymphoid organs

Stage IV Involvement of non-lymphoid organs such as liver, lung or bone marrow

Stage A   No symptoms meeting the criteria for stage B disease
Stage B   Having fever, drenching night sweats or significant weight loss (e.g. loss of more than 10% of body weight in the preceding 6 months)
The subscript E indicates that there is limited extranodal disease contiguous with known nodal disease.

Fig. 8.24. Staging of lymphoma.

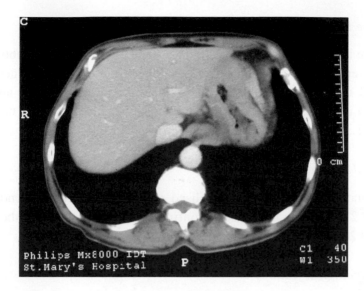

Fig. 8.25. Computed tomography (CT) scan of abdomen showing infiltration of the stomach by lymphoma. Gross thickening of the gastric wall is apparent.

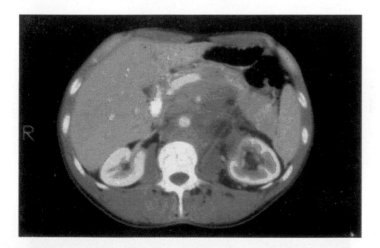

Fig. 8.26. CT scan of the abdomen after administration of oral and intravenous contrast medium. There is a mass of lymphomatous lymph nodes surrounding the aorta. Note that there is also hydronephrosis of the left kidney as a result of ureteric obstruction by the lymphoma.

Diffuse large B-cell lymphoma

Diffuse large B-cell lymphoma (DLBCL) is the most common subtype of NHL, representing about 40% of cases. It occurs at all ages. The neoplastic cell is a mature B cell but the cells are larger than normal and the disease is aggressive. A variety of translocations and mutations underlie DLBCL, which is actually quite a heterogeneous disease.

Clinical features

Presentation is usually with localised or generalised lymphadenopathy (Fig. 8.27). Sometimes disease is confined to the mediastinum or the brain (Fig. 8.28). B symptoms may be present.

Haematological features

The blood film and count are usually normal or show only non-specific features such as anaemia. Sometimes the bone marrow is infiltrated and, uncommonly, large lymphoma cells circulate in the blood.

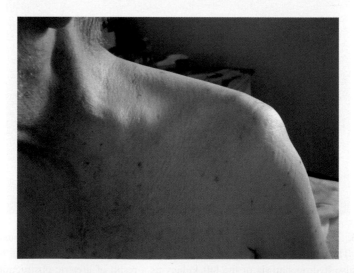

Fig. 8.27. Clinical photograph showing two enlarged lymph nodes in a patient with diffuse large B-cell lymphoma involving the left posterior triangle of the neck.

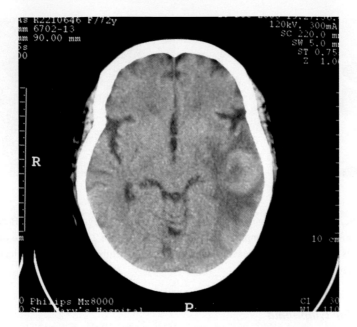

Fig. 8.28. CT scan of the head showing a lymphoma in the left cerebrum. The lymphoma occurred in a patient who had received immunosuppressive treatment and the lymphoma cells carried EBV.

Diagnosis and differential diagnosis

The diagnosis is usually made by lymph node biopsy. Sometimes a fine needle aspirate (Fig. 8.29) or a core needle biopsy permits a diagnosis. Immunohistochemistry or immunocytochemistry is needed to confirm that the neoplastic cells are B cells.

Management

Unless the disease is very localised and can be treated by radiotherapy, treatment is usually with combination chemo-immunotherapy, using the CHOP-R regime (cyclophosphamide, doxorubicin, vincristine, prednisolone and rituximab) and usually continuing for about 6 months. About 60% of patients can be cured.

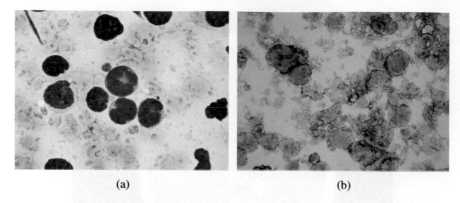

(a)   (b)

Fig. 8.29. Fine needle aspirate of a lymph node involved by diffuse large B-cell lymphoma showing: (a) large lymphoma cells (note that they are 2–3 times the size of the red blood cells); and (b) positive reaction on immunocytochemistry for CD20 indicating that the cells are of B lineage.

Follicular lymphoma

Follicular lymphoma is the second most common B-cell lymphoma representing about 25% of cases of NHL. The cell is a mature B cell related to a normal follicle centre cell and the neoplastic cells show a follicular growth pattern. This is a low-grade lymphoma. Disease is usually widespread (stage III or IV) at diagnosis. Follicular lymphoma results from a translocation in which the *BCL2* gene from chromosome 18 is dysregulated by being brought into proximity to the immunoglobulin heavy chain locus. Less often there is a translocation that results in *BCL2* being dysregulated by proximity to the kappa or lambda light chain locus.

Clinical features

Presentation is usually with lymphadenopathy and sometimes there is also splenomegaly. B symptoms may be present.

Haematological features

The blood film and count may be normal or there may be circulating lymphoma cells, sometimes in large numbers. These resemble normal

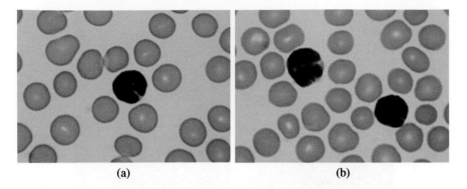

(a)   (b)

Fig. 8.30. PB film in follicular lymphoma showing small lymphoma cells with cleft nuclei.

follicle centre cells in that their nuclei are cleft (Fig. 8.30). The bone marrow is often infiltrated.

Diagnosis and differential diagnosis

Diagnosis is by lymph node biopsy, which demonstrates small cells with cleft nuclei with a follicular growth pattern (Fig. 8.31). Immunohistochemistry is essential to make a reliable distinction from reactive follicular hyperplasia as a response to antigenic stimulation. In follicular lymphoma, BCL2 is expressed by the cells that form follicles while in reactive hyperplasia it is not. Bone marrow infiltration is characteristically adjacent to the bone (paratrabecular).

In patients with circulating lymphoma cells the diagnosis can be made from the peripheral blood, using a combination of cytology, immunophenotyping and FISH analysis to demonstrate a translocation involving the *BCL2* gene.

Management

Occasionally, follicular lymphoma is localised and can be cured by radiotherapy. When it is generalised, cure is only possible with autologous stem cell transplantation but long survival can be achieved with chemoimmunotherapy, usually using a regime that is somewhat less intense

Fig. 8.31. Section of lymph node biopsy specimen from a patient with follicular lymphoma showing a follicular growth pattern.

than that used in DLBCL. In frail or elderly patients radiotherapy or single agent chemotherapy can achieve palliation and possibly prolongation of life.

T-cell lymphomas

T-cell lymphomas are less common than B-cell lymphomas. They are a heterogeneous group of diseases that are generally incurable, ranging from very-low grade to highly aggressive. Some show a predilection for the skin (Sézary syndrome and mycosis fungoides) while others involve lymph nodes or commence in the spleen or the gastrointestinal tract (enteropathy-associated T-cell lymphoma associated with coeliac disease). One distinctive unusual subtype is adult T-cell leukaemia/ lymphoma (ATLL) associated with infection with the human T-cell lymphotropic virus I (HTLVI).

Clinical features

Presentation varies from a chronic rash to a highly aggressive disease with generalised lymphadenopathy and hepatosplenomegaly. In aggressive subtypes, such as ATLL, there may be meningeal infiltration. There may be systemic symptoms such as fever, sweats, weight loss and itch.

Haematological features

The blood film and count usually show only non-specific features. There may be reactive eosinophilia. In Sézary syndrome, large or small neoplastic cells with convoluted nuclei circulate in the blood. In a subtype known as large granular lymphocyte lymphoma there are circulating neoplastic cells that are cytologically quite similar to normal large granular lymphocytes. The majority of patients with ATLL also have circulating lymphoma cells, which are distinctive for their lobulated, sometimes flower-shaped nuclei. The bone marrow is often infiltrated in T-cell lymphomas but infiltration may be subtle so that immunohistochemistry is necessary for confirmation.

Diagnosis and differential diagnosis

The diagnosis is usually made by biopsy of lymph node, skin or other tissue. However, when there are circulating neoplastic cells, diagnosis is often possible from a combination of cytology and immunophenotyping. Serology for HTLVI should be performed when ATLL is a possibility (e.g. in patients with typical haematological features and in patients with T-cell lymphoma originating in Japan, the Caribbean or other areas endemic for the virus).

Management

Management is very variable, depending on the specific subtype of lymphoma. Skin lymphomas may be effectively treated by therapy directed at the skin. Other T-cell lymphomas require systemic chemotherapy, usually combination chemotherapy. However, large granular lymphocyte leukaemia responds to oral methotrexate. ATLL shows some response to intensive chemotherapy and also to zidovudine plus interferon alpha but survival is nevertheless poor. Rituximab is of no use in T-cell lymphomas but immunotherapy with alemtuzumab, a monoclonal antibody directed at the CD52 antigen on T cells and other leucocytes, is of value in some subtypes.

Hodgkin Lymphoma

Hodgkin lymphoma (HL), also known as Hodgkin's disease, constitutes a separate category from NHL partly for historical reasons. Although the disease was first described in the 19th century it is only in recent decades that it has been possible to demonstrate its B-cell origin. It has been retained as a separate category because its histology and biological behaviour are distinctive. HL is divided into nodular lymphocyte-predominant HL, which is closer in nature to B-lineage NHL, and classical HL. Only classical HL will be discussed. This disease occurs at all ages, in Western countries from adolescence onwards but earlier in developing countries. There are strong aetiological links to EBV and there is a clear increase in EBV-related cases in patients with HIV infection.

Clinical features

Presentation is usually with lymphadenopathy although when disease is confined to the mediastinum the presenting feature may be cough. Systemic symptoms are common and in addition to the recognised B symptoms may include both itch and pain induced by alcohol consumption.

Haematological features

Anaemia with the features of anaemia of chronic disease is common; there may be eosinophilia and the erythrocyte sedimentation rate is raised. Except in HIV-related cases, bone marrow infiltration is uncommon.

Diagnosis and differential diagnosis

The diagnosis is made from histological examination following biopsy of a lymph node or other tissue. Hodgkin lymphoma is unusual in that the neoplastic cells are only a minority of cells in the involved tissue, the majority being polyclonal lymphocytes, eosinophils, fibroblasts and other reactive cells. The neoplastic cells are distinctive large mononuclear cells with large nucleoli (Hodgkin cells) or large binucleated or polylobated

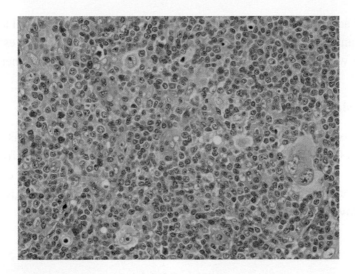

Fig. 8.32. Section of lymph node biopsy specimen from a patient with Hodgkin lymphoma showing a giant binucleated Reed–Sternberg cell (right) and several mononuclear Hodgkin cells. Note the characteristic large eosinophilic nucleoli in both the Reed–Sternberg cell and the mononuclear Hodgkin cells. The background cells are mainly lymphocytes and eosinophils.

cells, also with large nucleoli (Reed–Sternberg cells; Fig. 8.32). Immunohistochemistry is important in the diagnosis. Although the neoplastic cells are of B-cell origin they often fail to express common B-cell antigens whereas they express CD30 and usually CD15.

Management

Staging is of critical importance in determining the optimal treatment of HL. This is based on history, physical examination and CT scanning of chest abdomen and pelvis. A role for PET scanning at diagnosis has not yet established. A bone marrow biopsy is not generally needed, although in HIV-positive patients it may be the tissue that leads to the initial diagnosis of HL. Stage I and II HL can usually be cured with radiotherapy but because of the possible long-term sequelae of radiotherapy there is now a move to combining combination chemotherapy with more limited radiotherapy in the hope of achieving the same satisfactory outcome with less potential toxicity. PET scanning has a role in reducing treatment to that which is essential. Patients with stage III and IV disease require combination chemotherapy.

Conclusions

Diagnosis and classification of leukaemias and lymphomas is highly complex (in fact a great deal more complex than it might appear from this chapter). However, an accurate and very precise diagnosis is essential since more specific treatment for a variety of sub-types is now resulting in improved outcome for patients.

Test Case 8.1

A 65-year-old man has a blood count and a biochemical screening following admission to hospital with a myocardial infarction. Unexpectedly his blood count shows a lymphocytosis. He is re-examined and no lymphadenopathy, hepatomegaly or splenomegaly is found so the blood count is repeated the next day. It shows: WBC of $49 \times 10^9/l$, neutrophil count $6.1 \times 10^9/l$, lymphocyte count $42 \times 10^9/l$, monocyte count $0.9 \times 10^9/l$. The Hb and platelet count are normal. Immunophenotyping is done with the following results:

Kappa 85% (weak expression), lambda 5% (moderate expression)
CD19 88%
CD2 (a T-cell marker) 10%
CD5 94%
CD23 82%
FMC7 negative
CD79b negative

Questions

1. What is the most likely diagnosis and why?
2. Does the patient need any treatment for this condition at present?

You may wish to consult Table 8.2. Write down your answers before checking the correct answer (page 325) and re-reading any other relevant part of the chapter.

Test Case 8.2

A 4-year-old child is noted to be pale and listless by his mother. He is an only child and has previously been well. His GP finds him to have abdominal enlargement, lymphadenopathy and bruising and refers him urgently to hospital. An FBC shows: WBC of $146 \times 10^9/l$, neutrophil count $1.3 \times 10^9/l$, blast cells $144.7 \times 10^9/l$, Hb 8.7 g/dl and platelet count $86 \times 10^9/l$. The blast cells have no granules or Auer rods and are negative for myeloperoxidase and non-specific esterase and a blood sample is sent for immunophenotyping. A chest radiograph shows marked enlargement of the mediastinum.

Questions

1. What is the most likely diagnosis and why?
2. What other tests are needed?

Write down your answers before checking the correct answer (page 326) and re-reading any relevant part of the chapter.

9

Polycythaemia, Thrombocytosis and the Myeloproliferative Neoplasms

What Do You Have to Know?

☞ The nature of the myeloproliferative and myelodysplastic/ myeloproliferative neoplasms

☞ Polycythaemia vera — its clinicopathological features, differential diagnosis and principles of management

☞ Essential thrombocythaemia — its clinicopathological features, differential diagnosis and principles of management

☞ Primary myelofibrosis — its clinicopathological features, differential diagnosis and principles of management

☞ Chronic myelomonocytic leukaemia — its clinicopathological features, differential diagnosis and principles of management

The Nature of the Myeloproliferative and Myelodysplastic/ Myeloproliferative Neoplasms

The myeloproliferative neoplasms (MPN), also known as myeloproliferative disorders, are chronic neoplasms derived from a mutated multipotent haemopoietic progenitor cell (or in some instances, such as in chronic myelogenous leukaemia, from a pluripotent lymphoid-myeloid stem cell). They are characterised by **effective** production of mature cells, at least in the early stages of the disease. The three most important of these disorders are polycythaemia vera (PV), essential thrombocythaemia (ET) and primary myelofibrosis (PMF). These three conditions are closely related, often showing the same molecular abnormalities. Chronic myelogenous leukaemia (discussed in Chapter 8) can also be viewed as an MPN but at a molecular level is unrelated. All these conditions show a greater or lesser tendency to transform into acute myeloid leukaemia (AML). In addition, PV and ET can evolve into post-polycythaemic and post-essential thrombocythaemia myelofibrosis, with possible further disease evolution to AML (Fig. 9.1).

The myelodysplastic syndromes (MDS) have been discussed in Chapter 6. They differ from the MPN in that haemopoiesis is **ineffective**. The bone marrow is usually hypercellular in both groups of disorders but in MDS there is increased death of haemopoietic cells in the bone marrow so that there is inadequate production of mature cells of one or more lineages. This is in contrast to the increased production of one or more types of mature cell in the MPN. However, there are some haematological neoplasms in which there is effective production of cells of one lineage whereas another lineage shows ineffective haemopoiesis, which is often also morphologically dysplastic. For example, there could be a marked

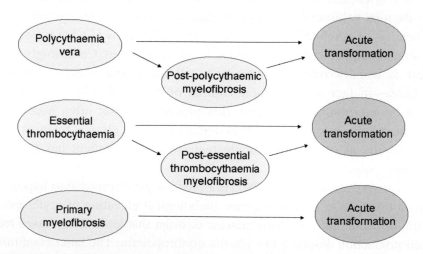

Fig. 9.1.   The possible disease course in polycythaemia vera, essential thrombocythaemia and primary myelofibrosis.

elevation of the platelet count associated with a sideroblastic anaemia or marked monocytosis associated with neutropenia. This group of disorders are designated myelodysplastic/myeloproliferative neoplasms (MDS/MPN).

Polycythaemia

Polycythaemia refers to an increase in the red cell count (RBC), haemoglobin concentration (Hb) and haematocrit (Hct) above what is normal for an individual of the same age and gender. These changes can indicate a true polycythaemia, meaning that the total volume of red cells in the bloodstream is increased, or a pseudopolycythaemia or apparent polycythaemia, meaning that there is a reduction in the plasma volume. To reliably distinguish between the two it is necessary to do isotopic dilution studies. The patient's red cells are labelled with a radioactive isotope such as ^{99m}Tc while the plasma is labelled by the addition of human albumin labelled with another radioactive isotope, such as ^{131}I or ^{125}I. A mixture of the labelled red cells and labelled plasma is then re-injected after first calculating the volume of red cells, volume of plasma and dose of each isotope that is to be injected. Taking blood samples from the patient after there has been time for mixing to occur permits a calculation of the total volume of red cells and plasma in which the re-injected specimen has been diluted. Results are expressed in terms of what is normal for an individual of the same gender, height and weight. Confusingly, this test is usually referred to as 'red cell mass and plasma volume' whereas in fact it is the total volume of both red cells and plasma that is determined. In practice, this procedure is not often necessary because it is generally possible to deduce from the clinical features and the results of other more simple tests whether a patient has true or pseudo-polycythaemia.

True polycythaemia can be: (i) a physiological response to hypoxia; (ii) a response to an inappropriate pathological elevation of erythropoietin; or (iii) an intrinsic bone marrow disorder that leads to increased red cell production despite a low plasma erythropoietin. The latter condition is called polycythaemia vera or polycythaemia rubra vera. Polycythaemia can be classified as primary or secondary (Box 9.1).

Box 9.1
Classification of polycythaemia

Primary — intrinsic bone marrow disease (polycythaemia vera)
Secondary — normal bone marrow response to an extrinsic stimulus
(either physiologically appropriate or inappropriate)

Polycythaemia that results from hypoxia can be beneficial since more oxygen can be delivered to tissues. However, if the Hct rises above 0.60 l/l there is a steep rise in whole blood viscosity, which can impair blood flow and therefore tissue oxygenation. Polycythaemia that results from inappropriate erythropoietin synthesis or intrinsic bone marrow disease is never beneficial and can be harmful since blood flow is impaired. Some of the more common causes of polycythaemia are summarised in Table 9.1.

Diagnostic approach to polycythaemia

A high Hb and Hct may be discovered incidentally or following presentation of a patient with relevant clinical features. The first essentials are a clinical history and physical examination. A clinical history should include personal history (e.g. of lung or renal disease), family history (e.g. of polycythaemia), drug history (diuretics, androgens) and smoking history. Symptoms suggestive of hypoxic lung disease should be sought. Physical examination may reveal splenomegaly, a renal mass, cyanosis, finger clubbing or features of chronic obstructive pulmonary disease (COPD).

The history and physical examination may reveal the likely cause, in which case further investigations can be focussed. For example, a patient with a history of smoking excess and with dyspnoea and an over-expanded hyper-resonant chest is likely to have COPD and a chest radiograph and arterial gas measurements are indicated whereas a patient presenting with thrombosis and found to have splenomegaly would be investigated immediately for polycythaemia vera. A family history of polycythaemia or detection at an unusually young age is an

Chapter 9

Table 9.1.   Some causes of polycythaemia.

	Mechanism		Possible causes
Apparent polycythaemia	Loss of plasma from the circulation or altered venous tone	Acute	Dehydration Shock Burns
		Chronic	Cigarette smoking Diuretics Unknown
True polycythaemia	Increased erythropoietin synthesis as a response to hypoxia		Living at a high altitude Hypoxic lung disease (e.g. chronic obstructive pulmonary disease, primary pulmonary hypertension) Cyanotic congenital heart disease Cigarette smoking (high carboxyhaemoglobin) High-affinity haemoglobin
	Inappropriately increased erythropoietin secretion		Renal cysts and tumours Renal artery stenosis Other tumours (rarely; e.g. hepatoma, cerebellar haemangioblastoma, phaeochromocytoma, uterine fibroids) Administration of androgens or related drugs Inappropriate use of erythropoietin (e.g. by athletes)
	Intrinsic bone marrow disease		Polycythaemia vera

indication to investigate for a high-affinity haemoglobin. If no likely cause is apparent from the history and physical examination, useful investigations may include: red cell mass and plasma volume; serum erythropoietin concentration; ultrasound or computed tomography (CT) examination of kidneys and spleen; chest radiography; arterial gas measurements; and molecular analysis for a *JAK2* mutation (see below). However, thought must be given to shortcuts so that the most relevant and potentially diagnostic test is done first and unnecessary investigation is thus avoided.

Polycythaemia vera

Polycythaemia vera is an MPN characterised by an increased RBC, Hb and Hct with or without an increase in the white cell count (WBC) and platelet count. It is mainly a disease of the elderly. This condition is now known to result from an acquired mutation in the *JAK2* gene occurring in a multipotent haemopoietic progenitor cell, which leads to abnormal proliferation signals without the need for erythropoietin to bind to erythropoietin receptors. In about 90–95% of patients this is a point mutation, *JAK2* V617F, in exon 14 of the gene. In another 5% of patients there is a mutation in exon 12.

Clinical features

Patients with polycythaemia usually have a plethoric complexion with conjunctival injection. The most prominent clinical features result from impaired circulation and thrombosis; they include headache, dizziness, transient ischaemic attacks, stroke, peripheral gangrene (Fig. 9.2), myocardial infarction and venous thromboembolism. The spleen may be

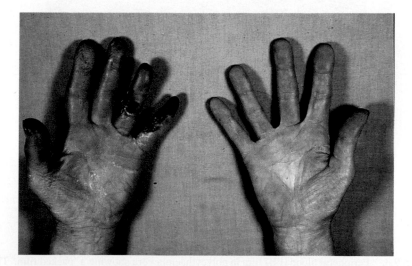

Fig. 9.2. Clinical photograph of the hands of a patient with polycythaemia vera showing poor circulation in the thumb and fingers of one hand with gangrene of two digits and impending gangrene of the others.

enlarged several cm below the left costal margin. Thrombosis of the hepatic vein can lead to hepatomegaly, jaundice and ascites (known as the Budd–Chiari syndrome). The portal vein and the mesenteric veins are also prone to thrombosis. There is an increased incidence of peptic ulceration and some patients suffer from itch, particularly after a hot bath; both of these clinical features result from increased histamine secretion by basophils. There is an increased incidence of gastrointestinal haemorrhage. Some patients suffer from gout since uric acid production is increased as a result of increased breakdown of nucleic acids.

Haematological features

Polycythaemia vera is characterised by an increased RBC, Hb and Hct and often also an increased WBC and neutrophil, basophil and platelet counts. The blood film has a 'packed' appearance as the increased viscosity of the blood makes it impossible to spread a thin film of blood on a glass slide (Fig. 9.3). The bone marrow is hypercellular as a result of

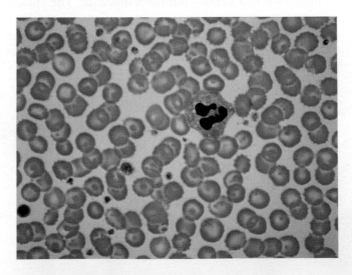

Fig. 9.3.   Peripheral blood (PB) film in polycythaemia vera showing a 'packed film.' The haemoglobin concentration (Hb) in this male patient was 20.2 g/dl and the haematocrit was 0.61 l/l. There is also thrombocytosis (platelet count 916×10^9/l) and some of the platelets are larger than normal. *JAK2* V617F was detected.

increased erythropoiesis. Granulopoiesis and megakaryocytes are usually also increased. Iron stores are usually absent as all the storage iron has been incorporated into the expanding red cell mass. Serum erythropoietin is low. Cytogenetic analysis may show a clonal cytogenetic abnormality, such as deletion of part of the long arm of chromosome 20, designated del(20q).

The blood count results may be confusing if there is complicating iron deficiency. The Hb and Hct may then be normal or low but the RBC is high and the WBC, platelet count and basophil count may be high.

Diagnosis and differential diagnosis

The diagnosis of polycythaemia vera used to require the measurement of red cell mass and plasma volume. Since the discovery of the very frequent presence of a *JAK2* mutation it is possible to base the diagnosis on the blood count plus mutational analysis. Only if there is clinically unexplained polycythaemia and no *JAK2* mutation is detected is it necessary to perform isotopic studies and then proceed to further investigations if a true polycythaemia is confirmed.

Management

It is necessary to correct the polycythaemia and any associated thrombocytosis. If there is isolated polycythaemia, the Hb and Hct can be lowered by regular venesection (of about 450 ml of blood on each occasion) until values are normal, followed by less frequent venesections to maintain normal values. Repeated venesection leads to depletion of iron stores so that infrequent venesection is then sufficient to maintain the Hct at a target value, e.g. less than 0.45 l/l or less than 0.50 l/l. Aspirin in a dose of 75 mg daily is prescribed to lessen the risk of thrombotic complications. Allopurinol may be needed. If the platelet count is also elevated the usual treatment is with an oral cytotoxic drug, hydroxycarbamide, plus aspirin. It is also possible to treat polycythaemia vera with a single injection of ^{32}P but this treatment increases the risk of transformation to acute leukaemia so is reserved for patients who are quite elderly or frail.

Some patients develop myelofibrosis or AML but nevertheless median survival with treatment is 10–20 years.

Thrombocytosis

Thrombocytosis (also referred to as thrombocythaemia) is an increase in the platelet count in comparison with the normal range for a person of the same age and gender. Thrombocytosis is a common non-specific reaction to infection and inflammation. Less often it is the result of an MPN, which in the case of isolated thrombocytosis is designated essential thrombocythaemia. Thrombocytosis may be primary or secondary (Box 9.2).

Box 9.2
Classification of thrombocytosis

Primary — intrinsic bone marrow disease (essential thrombocythaemia)
Redistributional — platelets redistributed from splenic pool into general circulation when the spleen has been removed or is atrophic
Secondary — normal bone marrow response to extrinsic stimulus

---

Some of the causes of thrombocytosis are shown in Table 9.2.

Essential thrombocythaemia

This is a haematological neoplasm resulting from mutation in a multipotent haemopoietic progenitor cell. In about half of cases the mutation is the same as that usually seen in polycythaemia vera, *JAK2* V617F. In another 5% of patients there is a mutation in the *MPL* gene that encodes the membrane receptor for thrombopoietin. In the remaining patients the precise nature of the mutation is not known. Essential thrombocythaemia occurs throughout adult life.

Clinical features

Diagnosis is often incidental, when a blood count is done for an unrelated condition or as part of a routine health check. Other patients present with

Table 9.2.   Some causes of thrombocytosis.

Mechanism	Cause
Reactive thrombocytosis	Infection
	Inflammation (e.g. inflammatory bowel disease, acute episodes in rheumatoid arthritis)
	Surgery or trauma
	Haemorrhage
	Haemolysis
	Malignant disease (e.g. carcinoma of lung)
	Iron deficiency
	Rebound following recovery from bone marrow suppression
Altered distribution of platelets	Post-splenectomy or hyposplenism
Intrinsic bone marrow disease	Essential thrombocythaemia
	Polycythaemia vera (many cases)
	Primary myelofibrosis (early stages of disease)
	Chronic myelogenous leukaemia (many cases)
	Myelodysplastic/myeloproliferative neoplasms (some cases)

either vascular insufficiency or thrombosis, e.g. with stroke or peripheral gangrene (Fig. 9.4). Microvascular involvement can lead to transient ischaemic attacks, disturbances of hearing and vision, recurrent headaches and erythromelalgia (burning pain, redness and warmth of the extremities). Paradoxically, patients with very high platelet counts may present with haemorrhage; the cause is the uptake of large multimers of von Willebrand factor by platelets, leading to acquired von Willebrand disease.

Haematological features

The blood film and count show thrombocytosis without polycythaemia (Fig. 9.5). Platelet size is increased. The WBC and neutrophil and basophil counts may be increased. The RBC, Hb and Hct are normal. The bone marrow shows an increase of megakaryocytes and these are larger than normal and form clusters. Erythropoiesis appears normal. Granulopoiesis may be increased. A minority of patients have a clonal cytogenetic abnormality.

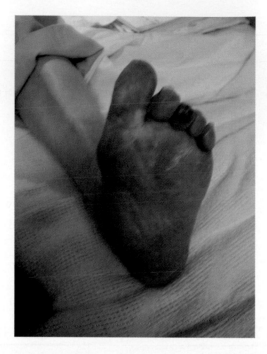

Fig. 9.4. Gangrene of the toes in a patient with essential thrombocythaemia.

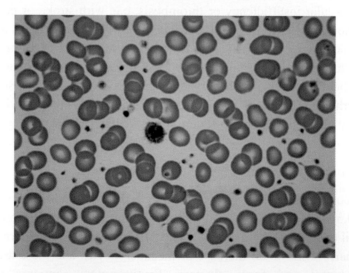

Fig. 9.5. PB film in a patient with essential thrombocythaemia showing thrombocytosis and one giant platelet. The platelet count was 1297×10^9/l with the white cell count, Hb and mean cell volume being normal.

Diagnosis and differential diagnosis

The diagnosis is most soundly based on demonstration of thrombocytosis with specific features supporting a diagnosis of an MPN, such as a *JAK2* or *MPL* mutation or a clonal cytogenetic abnormality. If evidence of clonality is absent, the diagnosis is made by exclusion of causes of reactive thrombocytosis and demonstration of typical bone marrow histology. If there is coexisting iron deficiency and a *JAK2* mutation, a diagnosis of PV cannot be excluded without the cautious administration of iron. The early stages of primary myelofibrosis can also be confused with ET, the distinction being based on bone marrow histology.

Management

In patients under the age of 60 years with only a moderate elevation of the platelet count (e.g. 400–1000 × 10^9/l) with no history of thrombosis there is no clear benefit from lowering the platelet count; these patients can be managed with aspirin 75 mg daily, to reduce the risk of thrombosis and, if they are smokers, they should be strongly advised to desist. In patients who are older or who have a higher count or a history of thrombosis, hydroxycarbamide to lower the platelet count is used together with aspirin. In patients with very marked thrombocytosis (e.g. a platelet count of 2000–3000 × 10^9/l), particularly with any history of bruising or haemorrhage, the count should be lowered by administering hydroxycarbamide before aspirin is given in order to avoid increasing the risk of haemorrhage. If patients cannot tolerate hydroxycarbamide, anagrelide can be substituted; it both lowers the platelet count and impairs platelet function so that aspirin can then be omitted.

Transformation to myelofibrosis or AML is quite infrequent and survival of patients with ET shows little reduction from normal.

Bone Marrow Fibrosis

Bone marrow fibrosis refers to the increased deposition of collagen and reticulin in the bone marrow. Sometimes there is an associated increase in bone deposition, known as osteosclerosis. Increased reticulin deposition is a very common non-specific abnormality; it should be distinguished from collagen fibrosis, which is associated with a more limited range of diagnoses. Some of the causes of collagen fibrosis are shown in Table 9.3.

Myelofibrosis can occur during the course of any of the MPN, but is crucial for the diagnosis of primary myelofibrosis.

Primary myelofibrosis

Primary myelofibrosis, sometimes called 'idiopathic myelofibrosis', is an MPN in which proliferation of a clone of cells derived from a mutated multipotent haemopoietic progenitor cell leads to reactive bone marrow fibrosis. In the early stages this may be reticulin fibrosis but in later stages there is extensive collagen deposition and sometimes osteosclerosis. It should be noted that the myelofibrosis is not really 'primary' as it is a response to cytokines secreted by neoplastic myeloid cells (particularly megakaryocytes). However, it is 'primary' in the sense that it occurs *de novo*, rather than following PV or ET. There is also mobilisation of haemopoietic progenitor cells from their niches in the bone marrow occurring early in the disease and leading to extramedullary haemopoiesis, particularly in the liver and spleen. A *JAK2* V617F mutation is present in about half of patients and an *MPL* mutation in about 15%. Clonal cytogenetic abnormalities are often present. Primary myelofibrosis is a disease of the middle-aged and elderly.

Table 9.3. **Some causes of collagen fibrosis of the bone marrow.**

Cause	Example
Myeloproliferative neoplasms	Primary myelofibrosis
	Post-polycythaemic myelofibrosis
	Post-essential thrombocythaemia myelofibrosis
	Chronic myelogenous leukaemia (rarely)
Acute myeloid leukaemia	Specific subtypes (e.g. acute megakaryoblastic leukaemia)
Lymphoma	Non-Hodgkin lymphoma
	Hodgkin lymphoma
Non-haemopoietic neoplasms	Metastatic carcinoma, particularly carcinoma of the breast or prostate
Bone diseases	Paget's disease, hyperparathyroidism, rickets, osteopetrosis (marble bone disease)

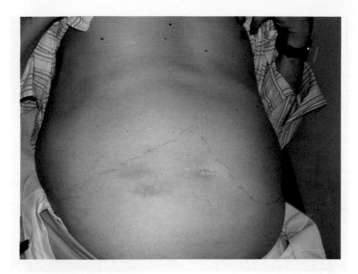

Fig. 9.6.   The abdomen of a patient with primary myelofibrosis with the size of the liver and spleen indicated. Note that there is also bruising.

Clinical features

Presentation is usually with hepatosplenomegaly, bruising and symptoms of anaemia (Figs. 9.6 and 9.7). The enlargement of the spleen may be very marked. There may be fatigue, weight loss, fever and increased sweating. Both haemorrhage and thrombosis can occur. In advanced disease, massive splenomegaly can cause hypersplenism, portal hypertension and ascites. Some patients suffer from gout.

Haematological features

In the early stages of the disease there may be thrombocytosis and an increased WBC. Later there is anaemia, leucopenia and thrombocytopenia. Cytopenias result from inadequate bone marrow production but, as progressive splenomegaly develops, hypersplenism plays a major role. The blood film is leucoerythroblastic (i.e. nucleated red blood cells and granulocyte precursors are present) and there are teardrop poikilocytes (Fig. 9.8). Because of the bone marrow fibrosis it may be impossible to aspirate bone marrow or there may be aspiration only of blood from bone

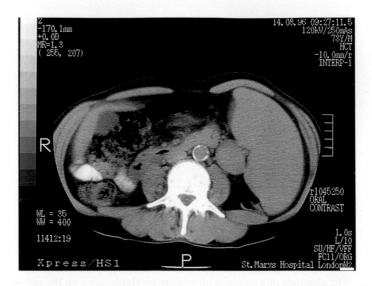

Fig. 9.7. Computed tomography (CT) scan of abdomen in a patient with primary myelofibrosis showing very marked splenomegaly. (There is also calcification in the wall of the aorta.)

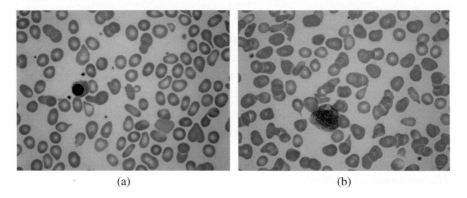

(a)   (b)

Fig. 9.8. PB film from a patient with primary myelofibrosis showing teardrop poikilocytes, elliptocytes, a nucleated red blood cell (a) and a myelocyte (b). Note that there are very few platelets.

marrow sinusoids. Diagnosis is dependent on trephine biopsy histology, which demonstrates the fibrosis (Fig. 9.9). Late in the course of the disease, haemopoiesis is ineffective and the lactate dehydrogenase is markedly elevated. Haemopoietic cells may be dysplastic.

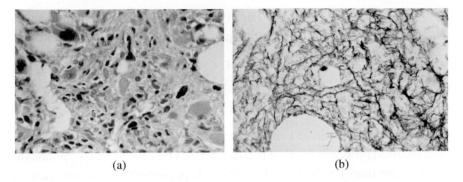

(a)   (b)

Fig. 9.9. Trephine biopsy sections from a patient with primary myelofibrosis showing (a) megakaryocytes and other haemopoietic cells embedded in pale pink collagen on a haematoxylin and eosin stain; (b) increased reticulin deposition on a reticulin stain.

Diagnosis and differential diagnosis

In advanced disease the diagnosis is straightforward, being based on clinical features, a leucoerythroblastic anaemia with teardrop poikilocytes and a fibrotic bone marrow. The clinical history permits a distinction from post-PV and post-ET myelofibrosis and bone marrow histology permits a distinction from other causes of bone marrow fibrosis.

Management

Management is difficult and generally unsatisfactory. Among the agents that are sometimes of benefit are hydroxycarbamide (for thrombocytosis or painful splenomegaly), danazol (an anabolic steroid) or erythropoietin (for anaemia) and thalidomide or lenalidomide. Patients with advanced disease may require blood transfusion and sometimes splenectomy or splenic irradiation. Allopurinol may be needed. Treatment offers only rather inadequate palliation. Median survival is about 5 years.

Myelodysplastic/Myeloproliferative Neoplasms

The MDS/MPN include chronic myelomonocytic leukaemia (CMML), atypical chronic myeloid leukaemia and a condition of children, juvenile myelomonocytic leukaemia. The Philadelphia chromosome and the *BCR-ABL1* fusion gene are absent. Only CMML will be discussed further, the other two conditions being rare.

Chronic myelomonocytic leukaemia

This is a chronic myeloid neoplasm resulting from mutation in a multipotent myeloid progenitor cell; it is characterised by monocytosis (monocyte count more than 1×10^9/l) and anaemia. It is predominantly a disease of the elderly. Transformation to AML can occur.

Clinical features

Presentation may be with symptoms of anaemia or with other systemic symptoms such as weight loss, fatigue and increased sweating. Some patients have infection or bleeding. Physical examination may show splenomegaly and, less often, hepatomegaly.

Haematological features

The blood count usually shows leucocytosis and anaemia and sometimes thrombocytopenia. There is monocytosis (Fig. 9.10). The neutrophil count may be high, normal or low. There may be anisocytosis and poikilocytosis and dysplastic changes in neutrophils (hypolobulation, hypogranularity). The bone marrow aspirate shows increased cellularity. Dysplastic features may include sideroblastic erythropoiesis. Blast cells may be increased in the blood and the bone marrow but are not as numerous as in AML (less than 20%). Cytogenetic analysis may show an acquired clonal abnormality, such as trisomy 8. The Philadelphia chromosome and t(9;22) is **not** found.

Diagnosis and differential diagnosis

The differential diagnosis is with a leukaemoid reaction due, for example, to infection and with other types of chronic myeloid leukaemia.

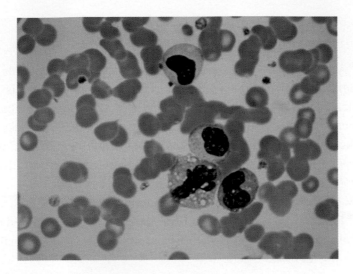

Fig. 9.10. PB film from a patient with chronic myelomonocytic leukaemia showing two monocytes (bottom) and two dysplastic neutrophils (top); the neutrophils are hypogranular with defective lobulation.

Management

Patients do not necessarily require treatment at diagnosis. If there are symptoms, blood transfusion and oral chemotherapy may be of benefit.

Conclusions

The myeloproliferative neoplasms are haematological neoplasms that produce their disease manifestations through overproduction of mature cells of one or more lineages. In the case of primary myelofibrosis, extra-medullary haemopoiesis, bone marrow fibrosis and progressive bone marrow failure are also characteristic. Chronic myelomonocytic leukaemia differs from the myeloproliferative neoplasms in also having dysplastic features. Polycythaemia vera and essential thrombocythaemia can be effec-tively treated whereas treatment of primary myelofibrosis and chronic myelomonocytic leukaemia is less satisfactory.

Test Case 9.1

A 73-year-old retired accountant presents with left hemiparesis and is found on CT scanning to have a right cerebral infarct. His past medical history is of a hernia repair and varicose veins. He takes no medications, drinks a glass of wine most evenings and does not smoke. On examination, he is noted to be plethoric. His blood pressure is normal. The spleen is not palpable. FBC shows: WBC $16.3 \times 10^9/l$ (normal range [NR] 3.7–9.5), Hb 19 g/dl (NR 13.3–16.7), MCV 85 fl (NR 82–98) and platelet count $582 \times 10^9/l$ (NR 168–411). The blood film shows a 'packed film' appearance and increased neutrophils and basophils. A *JAK2* V617F mutation is found on analysis of peripheral blood leucocytes.

Questions

1. What is the most likely cause of the stroke and the haematological abnormalities?
2. Are there any other essential tests?
3. What is the immediate management of the patient?
4. What is the long-term management?

Write down your answers before checking the correct answer (page 326) and re-reading any relevant part of the chapter.

10

Multiple Myeloma

What Do You Have to Know?

☞ The clinicopathological effects of multiple myeloma, when to suspect it, how it is diagnosed and the principles of treatment

☞ The nature and significance of monoclonal gammopathy of undetermined significance, how it is diagnosed

Introduction

In healthy people plasma cells are present in small numbers in many tissues. In the bone marrow they are normally about 1% of nucleated cells and are polyclonal — some expressing kappa light chain and some lambda.

Multiple myeloma, also know as plasma cell myeloma, is a neoplastic disorder of plasma cells that usually originates in the bone marrow and is widespread at diagnosis. Much less commonly a plasma cell neoplasm presents as a solitary tumour, arising either in the bone marrow or elsewhere. A solitary plasmacytoma occurring outside the bone marrow is referred to as an extramedullary plasmacytoma.

Multiple myeloma is usually associated with secretion of an abnormal immunoglobulin molecule known as a paraprotein. A paraprotein is also present though at a lower concentration in a neoplastic, but much more benign, condition known as monoclonal gammopathy of undetermined significance (MGUS). The presence of a paraprotein can also occur in other plasma cell and lymphoplasmacytic neoplasms (see below).

Multiple Myeloma

Multiple myeloma is a disease resulting from proliferation of neoplastic plasma cells in the bone marrow and other tissues. Often the plasma cells synthesise an immunoglobulin (Ig) molecule, either IgG, IgA or, uncommonly, IgD or IgE. Because this paraprotein is the product of a clone of cells it has a single light chain type, kappa or lambda. The monoclonal light chain may be synthesised in excess and as it has a low molecular weight it is excreted by the kidney. It is known as a Bence–Jones protein. In other cases of myeloma (about 20% of cases) the cells synthesise only light chain. This form of the disease is known as Bence–Jones myeloma. When there is renal failure, excretion of Bence–Jones protein is reduced and it may then be found in the blood in appreciable amounts. In a small minority of patients with myeloma (2–3%) the cells are so abnormal that they do not secrete appreciable amounts of immunoglobulin although it is detectable in the cytoplasm (non-secretory myeloma). Very rarely the cells do not synthesise any detectable immunoglobulin or immunoglobulin fragment (non-producing myeloma).

The clinicopathological features of multiple myeloma result from: (i) the direct effects of proliferation of the neoplastic cells, such as destruction of bone and pathological fractures; (ii) the indirect metabolic effects of the tumour, such as hyperuricaemia and hypercalcaemia; (iii) the damaging effects of the immunoglobulin molecule or the Bence–Jones protein, such as peripheral neuropathy or renal failure; (iv) the effects of amyloid deposition (which occurs in some patients, amyloid being formed from the monoclonal light chain); and (v) impaired immunity as a result of a reduction in the concentration of normal polyclonal immunoglobulins. Hypercalcaemia is the result of stimulation of osteoclast activity directly or indirectly by myeloma cells. Renal failure is common in myeloma and is multifactorial (Box 10.1).

> **Box 10.1**
> **Causes of renal failure in myeloma**
>
> Hypercalcaemia
> Hyperuricaemia
> Dehydration (may be due to hypercalcaemia)
> Damage to the kidney by Bence–Jones protein (protein casts within tubules and damage to tubular cells)
> Amyloidosis
> Infection
> Use of non-steroidal anti-inflammatory drugs for pain relief, nephrotoxic antibiotics or radiological contrast media

Clinical features

Multiple myeloma is the second most common haematological neoplasm after non-Hodgkin lymphoma with an incidence of about 5/100 000/year. This is predominantly a disease of the elderly with the median age of presentation being 65–70 years. Patients with multiple myeloma often present with bone pain or a pathological fracture. Back ache is common; vertebral collapse can cause acute back pain. Spinal cord compression may occur, either as a result of vertebral collapse or due to tumour growth adjacent to the spinal cord. Other patients present with symptoms of anaemia such as fatigue, lethargy and dyspnoea. Presentation can also be with renal failure or recurrent infection. A minority of patients with a very high paraprotein concentration have clinical features, such as blurred vision, resulting from hyperviscosity. Some patients are asymptomatic at diagnosis and the diagnosis is an incidental one. Patients who develop amyloidosis may have macroglossia, cardiac failure and nephrotic syndrome as well as renal failure.

Laboratory features

The blood count shows anaemia, which is either normocytic or macrocytic. There may be thrombocytopenia. Because of the high concentration of the paraprotein, the red cells form into rouleaux (Fig. 10.1) and the blood film stains abnormally blue, an appearance referred to as 'increased background staining'. When the paraprotein concentration is very high the blue staining may be visible macroscopically (Fig. 10.2). The increased

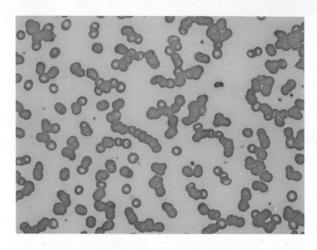

Fig. 10.1. Peripheral blood (PB) film in multiple myeloma showing increased rouleaux formation.

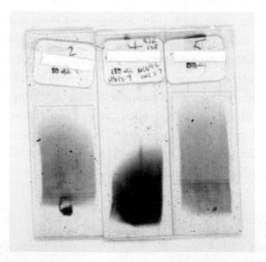

Fig. 10.2. Three blood films, the centre one from a patient with multiple myeloma, showing the intense blue colour of the stained film as a result of a high concentration of a paraprotein.

protein concentration also leads to an increase in the erythrocyte sedimentation rate (ESR). In patients with Bence–Jones or non-secretory myeloma there is no increase in plasma protein concentration and there is therefore no increase in rouleaux formation or background staining; the ESR is either normal or is mildly elevated as a consequence of the anaemia. In some patients there are neoplastic plasma cells in the circulation, usually in small numbers (Fig. 10.3). Rarely there are large numbers of circulating myeloma cells, referred to as plasma cell leukaemia.

Biochemical tests usually show an increased concentration of one immunoglobulin type and serum protein electrophoresis shows a discrete band (Fig. 10.4) which, on immunofixation can be identified as a paraprotein (i.e. having a single type of heavy chain and light chain; Fig. 10.5). The normal immunoglobulins are reduced. In patients with Bence–Jones myeloma or non-secretory myeloma all that will be detected on electrophoresis is a reduction of normal immunoglobulins but measurement of serum-free light chains (see below) shows an abnormality. Other biochemical abnormalities that may be present in the blood include increased urea, creatinine, uric acid or calcium. The alkaline phosphatase is usually normal.

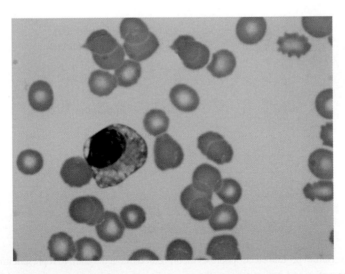

Fig. 10.3. PB film in multiple myeloma showing a myeloma cell and increased background staining.

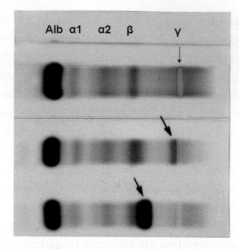

Fig. 10.4. Serum protein electrophoresis showing: (a) a normal sample showing albumin (Alb) and α1, α2, β and γ globulins; (b) sample from a patient with multiple myeloma showing a paraprotein band in the gamma region (black arrow); and (c) sample from a patient with multiple myeloma showing a paraprotein band in the beta region. The red arrow indicates the application point. Note that normal background γ globulins are reduced in the two myeloma samples.

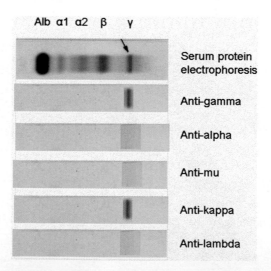

Fig. 10.5. Serum protein electrophoresis incorporated into a diagram to represent immunofixation. With anti-γ and anti-κ antisera there is a discrete band corresponding to the band on electrophoresis showing the presence of an IgGκ paraprotein. With anti-α, anti-μ and anti-λ antisera there is diffuse staining representing the background polyclonal immunoglobulins.

Biochemical tests of urine may show the presence of a Bence–Jones protein. Initially, this free monoclonal light chain was detected by abnormal characteristics on heating; it coagulates at 45° to 55°C but redissolves on heating to a higher temperature. Nowadays, this protein is detected by electrophoresis and immunofixation of a concentrated (early morning) urine sample. The urine may also contain albumin.

Diagnosis

Diagnosis is usually based on clinical suspicion leading to a blood count and film, measurement of the ESR, and electrophoresis and immunofixation of both serum and urine. It must be remembered that diagnosis is more difficult in patients with Bence–Jones myeloma because of the lack of the usual blood film features and the lack of an elevated ESR. Diagnosis is even more difficult in the uncommon cases of non-secretory or non-producing myeloma. An alternative to detection of urinary Bence–Jones protein as a screening test for Bence–Jones myeloma is a measurement of free light chains in the serum. This immunological assay detects the very small amount of free monoclonal light chains that are present in the serum in healthy people and to a greater extent in the great majority of patients with multiple myeloma; detection of an excess of either kappa or lambda light chains is a sensitive test for myeloma, including Bence–Jones myeloma and non-secretory myeloma.

A bone marrow aspirate is essential for diagnosis and usually shows 10–90% of plasma cells, which are often cytologically abnormal (Figs. 10.6–10.8). They may be pleomorphic, larger than normal or multi-nucleated, and may contain round or linear immunoglobulin inclusions. Low plasma cell numbers in an aspirate may be because the infiltration is initially focal; because of associated fibrosis, the plasma cells may also be more resistant to aspiration than normal bone marrow cells. For these reasons a trephine needle biopsy, in which a core of bone and bone marrow is obtained, is more sensitive that a bone marrow aspirate in detecting and quantitating infiltration by multiple myeloma. Cytogenetic analysis of plasma cells may disclose a clonal chromosomal abnormality, the precise abnormality found being of prognostic significance.

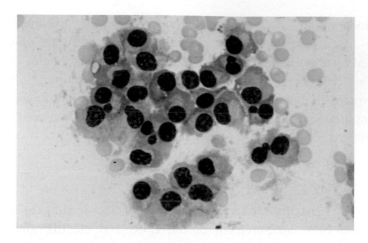

Fig. 10.6. Bone marrow (BM) aspirate film from a patient with multiple myeloma showing that normal haemopoietic cells have been replaced by myeloma cells. The basophilic cytoplasm, eccentric nucleus and pale paranuclear Golgi zone identify the cells as plasma cells but note that many of them have nuclei of abnormal shapes. Low power.

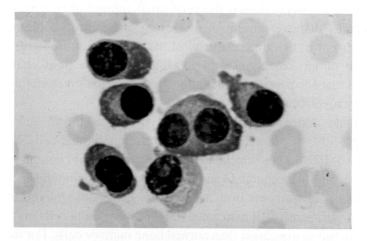

Fig. 10.7. BM aspirate film from a patient with multiple myeloma showing myeloma cells. There is one binucleate cell and one cell (beneath the binucleate cell) that has a nucleolus. High power.

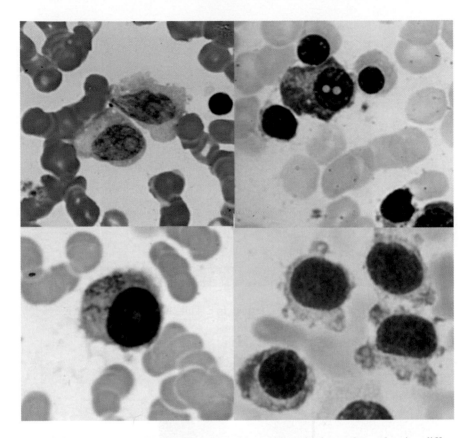

Fig. 10.8. BM aspirate films from four patients with multiple myeloma showing different cytological abnormalities: plasmablasts, showing a lack of chromatin condensation and nucleoli (top left); globules of immunoglobulin overlying nucleus (top right); cytoplasmic granules and crystals in a nucleolated myeloma cell (bottom left); and plasma cells with a high nucleocytoplasmic ration and cytoplasmic blebs.

A skeletal survey is important in diagnosis and management. The most distinctive abnormality is the presence of multiple punched out lytic lesions in the skull (Fig. 10.9). Other bones may also show lytic lesions (Fig. 10.10) and sometimes these are extensive (Fig. 10.11). The vertebral column may either have changes resembling osteoporosis or may show discrete lytic lesions; vertebral collapse may be demonstrated. Occasionally, there is

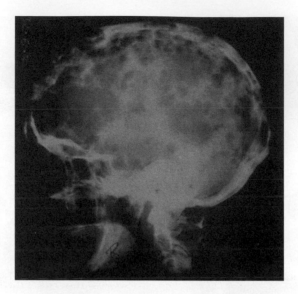

Fig. 10.9. Punched out lytic lesions in a skull radiograph in myeloma.

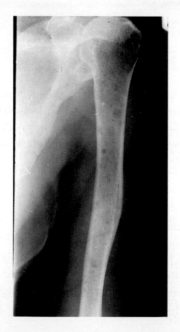

Fig. 10.10. Small lytic lesions in a radiograph of the humerus in multiple myeloma.

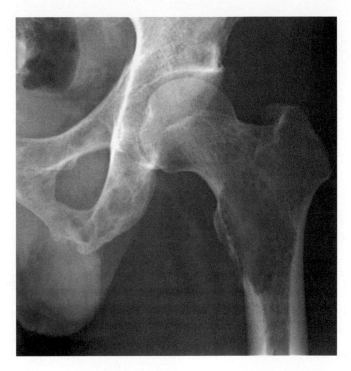

Fig. 10.11. Radiograph of the hip and part of the pelvis showing an extensive lytic lesion extending from the neck into the shaft of the femur. There are smaller lytic lesions in the pubic ramus.

sclerosis of bone. Computed tomography scanning is also useful for showing the extent of bony lesions (Fig. 10.12).

Other essential tests include quantification of any serum paraprotein, quantification of Bence–Jones protein in a 24-hour urine collection, measurement of calcium, phosphate, alkaline phosphatase and uric acid, and assessment of liver and renal function. Alkaline phosphatase is usually normal but may be increased if there are osteosclerotic lesions or healing fractures. Beta$_2$ microglobulin is measured since a high concentration correlates with a worse prognosis. Other adverse prognostic factors are: more severe anaemia, the presence of a Bence–Jones protein, elevated creatinine, a higher paraprotein concentration, a lower albumin concentration, hypercalcaemia and extensive skeletal lesions.

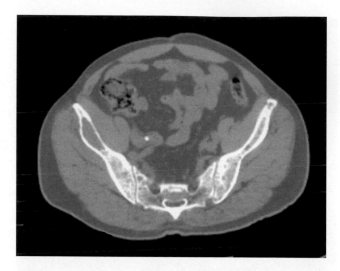

Fig. 10.12.   Computed tomography (CT) scan showing lytic lesions in the pelvis and sacrum.

Management

It is necessary to investigate carefully to distinguish multiple myeloma from MGUS and also to distinguish asymptomatic myeloma (which requires observation but not treatment) from symptomatic myeloma (which requires treatment). 'Symptomatic myeloma' includes patients with end-organ damage as well as those with symptoms. Asymptomatic myeloma is distinguished from MGUS (see below) by having **either** a paraprotein present at a concentration of more than 30 g/l or more than 10% of clonal plasma cells in the bone marrow.

Treatment is both supportive and directed specifically at the plasma cell neoplasm. Supportive treatment may include red cell transfusions for anaemia and antibiotic treatment for any infection. Patients with hypercalcaemia require re-hydration, corticosteroids and a bisphosphonate. Regular bisphosphonates (pamidronate, clodronate or zoledronic acid) can be prescribed in these and other patients and their use is associated with less pain, fewer pathological fractures and better survival. Allopurinol may be needed. Patients with renal insufficiency may require dialysis, which will also correct life-threatening hyperkalaemia. If renal failure is due to the damaging effects of Bence–Jones proteins, dialysis is urgent; special membranes are available that permit removal of light chains. Chemotherapy should be introduced promptly in such patients in order to reduce light chain production rapidly. Unless dialysis and early chemotherapy are employed, renal failure may be irreversible. Patients who have suffered a pathological fracture can benefit from pinning the fracture plus local radiotherapy.

A considerable number of chemotherapeutic agents are now available for the treatment of multiple myeloma. Depending on the age and general health of the patients, these range from single agent oral chemotherapy (with melphalan) to intensive combination chemotherapy followed by autologous stem cell transplantation. This is generally applicable in patients under the age of 50 years, but sometimes even up to the age of 70 years. The latter improves survival in comparison with less intensive treatment and is considered the treatment of choice if the patient is fit enough. Effective cytotoxic and other agents in myeloma include alkylating agents (melphalan, cyclophosphamide), vinca alkaloids (vincristine), anthracyclines (doxorubicin), corticosteroids (prednisolone or dexamethasone), immune modulating agents (interferon alpha, thalidomide, lenalidomide), antiangiogenesis agents (thalidomide, lenalidomide) and proteasome inhibitors (bortezomib). Although these various agents, often in combination, can induce remission and improve survival, the only potentially curative treatment is allogeneic stem cell transplantation.

Median survival was previously 3–4 years. Autologous stem cell transplantation has extended this to around 5 years and the use of newly introduced agents such as lenalidomide and bortezomib may have extended it further, probably up to 6 years.

Monoclonal Gammopathy of Undermined Significance

MGUS describes the presence of a low concentration monoclonal immunoglobulin (usually IgG, IgA or IgM) in the blood without any clinical or pathological evidence of associated disease. There is an associated increase in monoclonal plasma cells in the bone marrow. MGUS is found in about 1% of adults, increasing to a prevalence of 2% over the age of 50 years, 2–4% in people in their 60s, 4–5% in people in their 70s and 14% over the age of 90 years. Since there are no clinical manifestations this is necessarily a diagnosis that is made incidentally when patients are being investigated for an unrelated condition. In the majority of instances, the individual with MGUS remains free of associated disease. However, evolution to multiple myeloma occurs in about 1% of patients per year (one-quarter of patients by 25 years from initial detection). Evolution to non-Hodgkin lymphoma and development of amyloidosis are other possible outcomes.

Clinical features

There are no clinical features.

Laboratory features

A serum paraprotein is present but at a concentration of 30 g/l or less.

Diagnosis

Diagnosis is based on detection of a low concentration paraprotein on serum protein electrophoresis and immunofixation. A bone marrow aspiration is not usually indicated but if it is performed the plasma cells may be up to 10% whereas in the marrow of a healthy person they are around 1%. Similar numbers of plasma cells may be found in patients with a variety of infective and inflammatory conditions but these are polyclonal (some cells expressing κ light chains and some expressing λ).

Management

No treatment is indicated. In the elderly follow-up may not even be indicated. Younger patients can have investigations repeated at 6-month to yearly intervals, depending on the concentration of the paraprotein, as long as they remain asymptomatic.

Other Conditions Associated with Paraproteinaemia

Paraproteins can also be detected in other B-lineage neoplasms in which there is differentiation to plasmacytoid lymphocytes or plasma cells (Table 10.1). They are detected in some patients with non-Hodgkin lymphoma, particularly but not only lymphoplasmacytoid lymphoma. Some such patients have a high concentration of an IgM paraprotein with associated clinical features due to hyperviscosity. This condition is known as Waldenström macroglobulinaemia. Other patients with an IgM paraprotein have cryoglobulinaemia (Fig. 10.13) or cold agglutinin disease.

Light chain-associated (AL) amyloidosis can occur in association with multiple myeloma or non-Hodgkin lymphoma or can be a primary

Table 10.1. **Other conditions associated with a paraprotein.**

Condition	Possible clinical effects
Lymphoplasmacytic and other non-Hodgkin lymphoma	Hyperviscosity, cryoglobulinaemia, cold-induced haemolysis (chronic cold haemagglutinin disease)
Light chain-associated (AL) amyloidosis	Nephrotic syndromes and renal failure, cardiac failure, macroglossia, peripheral neuropathy
Light chain deposition disease	Nephrotic syndrome or renal failure
Heavy chain diseases	Variable

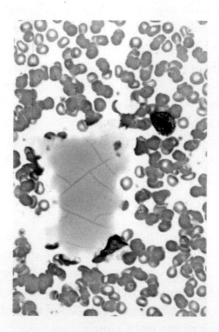

Fig. 10.13. PB film showing a large deposit of cryoglobulin, which precipitated as the blood cooled *in vitro*.

disease with bone marrow clonal plasma cell numbers being present in low numbers.

Conclusions

Multiple myeloma and monoclonal gammopathy of undetermined significance (MGUS) are both plasma cell neoplasms but with differing clinical significance. Both are characterised by the presence of a paraprotein. Paraproteins can also be present in other patients with neoplasms of plasma cells or lymphoplasmacytoid lymphocytes. Sometimes a paraprotein is a marker of the disease but is in itself harmless. In other patients, paraproteins cause a variety of clinical manifestations and tissue damage of diverse types.

Test Case 10.1

A 57-year-old housewife develops a painful left shoulder and notices that it appears swollen. She does not remember having injured it. Her GP arranges an X-ray, which shows a lytic lesion expanding the lateral end of the left clavicle. He notices that she is also quite pale and refers her to Haematology outpatients. There she is found to be anaemic, the FBC showing WBC 7.8×10^9/l, Hb 9.5 g/dl (normal range [NR] 11.8–14.8), MCV 106 fl (NR 82–98) and platelet count 102×10^9/l. The ESR is 74 mm in one hour (NR 0–20). Serum vitamin B_{12} and red cell folate assays are normal. An IgAκ paraprotein is detected in a concentration of 36 g/dl but Bence–Jones protein is not detected. A bone marrow aspirate shows 13% plasma cells.

Question

Consider the information that you have been given in this chapter and work out if the patient has extramedullary myeloma, symptomatic myeloma, asymptomatic myeloma, MGUS or something else. **Write down your answers before checking the correct answer (page 327) and re-reading any relevant parts of the chapter if you did not come to the right conclusion.**

11

Platelets, Coagulation and Haemostasis

What Do You Have to Know?

☞ How haemostasis is achieved

☞ The function of the platelet

☞ How coagulation is controlled and blood clots are lysed

☞ The coagulation cascade *in vivo* and *in vitro*

☞ How to interpret coagulation screening tests

☞ The clinicopathological features and diagnosis of the most common inherited defects of coagulation

☞ The clinicopathological features and diagnosis of common acquired defects of coagulation

☞ The principles of treatment of coagulation abnormalities

☞ The causes, investigation and management of thrombocytopenia including autoimmune thrombocytopenic purpura and thrombotic thrombocytopenic purpura

Overview of Haemostasis

When the vessel wall is damaged or breached the blood is exposed to molecules that initiate the process of haemostasis or coagulation, resulting in the formation of a stable clot that prevents death from haemorrhage. At the same time, processes that ultimately dissolve the clot are initiated

217

and healing commences. Intricate anticoagulant mechanisms are also activated and prevent propagation of the clot away from the area of damage; obstruction of blood flow in other vessels is thus prevented. The haemostatic process can be usefully divided into primary and secondary haemostasis, although in fact they are initiated and progress more or less simultaneously.

Primary haemostasis — platelets

Breach of the vessel wall exposes collagen and other elements of the extracellular matrix to which plasma, von Willebrand factor (VWF) and platelets will bind, a process enhanced by the shear stress of blood flow. VWF binding to collagen facilitates binding of more platelets. During the process of binding, platelets become activated, releasing adenosine diphosphate (ADP), thromboxane A2 and VWF so that additional platelets are captured and activated. The result is formation of the primary platelet plug which blocks further loss of blood.

Secondary haemostasis — coagulation

Blood escaping from the area of damage is exposed to tissue factor which is expressed at high levels on cells surrounding the vessel, forming what has been called a 'haemostatic envelope'. Tissue factor binds to factor VII in plasma, forming an activated complex and thus blood coagulation is initiated. This is called the 'extrinsic pathway' because tissue factor is regarded as extrinsic to the blood. It is the physiological pathway for coagulation activation *in vivo*. The tissue factor-factor VII complex converts factor X into its active form (Xa) by proteolytic cleavage and Xa is now able to convert a small amount of prothrombin (factor II) into thrombin, again by proteolytic cleavage (Fig 11.1). A crucial action of this thrombin is to activate the two co-factors, factor V and factor VIII into their active forms: factor VIIIa and factor Va are not enzymes but greatly increase the activity of the enzymes factor IXa (also activated by the tissue factor-factor VII complex) and factor Xa by approximately five orders of magnitude. The result is a major amplification of the original stimulus and an enormous burst of thrombin generation (Fig. 11.2). The final stage

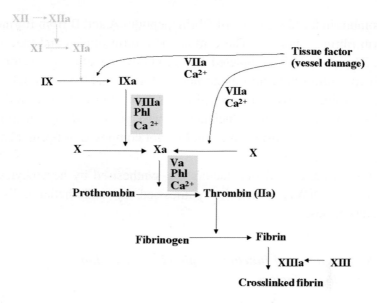

Fig. 11.1. The first steps of *in vivo* coagulation. Phl = phospholipid provided by activated platelets.

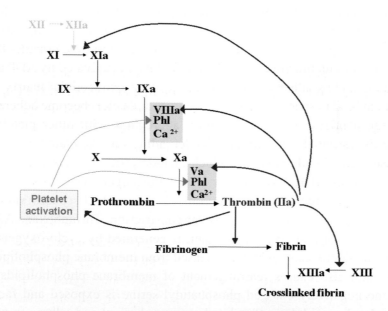

Fig. 11.2. Enhancement of *in vivo* coagulation by thrombin that is generated (red arrows) and by activated platelets (green arrows). It will be seen that factor XII has no role in *in vivo* coagulation. Phl = phospholipid provided by activated platelets.

is thrombin-induced cleavage of fibrinopeptides A and B from fibrinogen to form fibrin monomers. These monomers form dimers and then polymers. The process is completed by thrombin activation of factor XIII which cross-links the fibrin monomers to form a stable clot. Soluble fibrinogen is thus converted into stable insoluble fibrin. Fibrin binds and stabilises the platelet plug, which is otherwise prone to disaggregation, so that finally there is a firm and insoluble clot composed of fibrin, platelets and other blood cells.

Most of the coagulation factors are synthesised by hepatocytes. An exception is VWF, which is synthesised by endothelial cells and megakaryocytes.

Platelet structure and function — platelet interaction with coagulation factors

Platelets are formed in the bone marrow by fragmentation of megakaryocyte cytoplasm, the platelets entering the circulating blood when they are shed into bone marrow sinusoids. Each megakaryocyte can produce about 4000 platelets. Platelets survive in the circulation for about 10 days. The platelet has surface receptors and cytoplasmic granules that are crucial to its function (Fig. 11.3). Platelets are activated by ADP and thrombin and by adhesion to constituents of the extracellular matrix, all of which bind to specific receptors. Activated platelets become adherent, undergo a release reaction and form aggregates with other platelets. VWF is essential for normal platelet adhesion. Activated platelets release their granule contents, which include procoagulants and aggregants such as ADP, VWF, factor V and fibrinogen. They also release serotonin (previously taken up from plasma), which causes smooth muscle contraction and thus arteriolar constriction. Thromboxane A2, a vasoconstrictor and potent aggregant, is generated by cyclo-oxygenase from arachidonic acid, which is released from membrane phospholipids. Activation also causes rearrangement of membrane phospholipids so that the negatively charged phosphatidyl serine is exposed and facilitates blood coagulation. Platelets become spherical and adhere to each other forming a loose platelet plug, which is also adherent to the site of tissue damage.

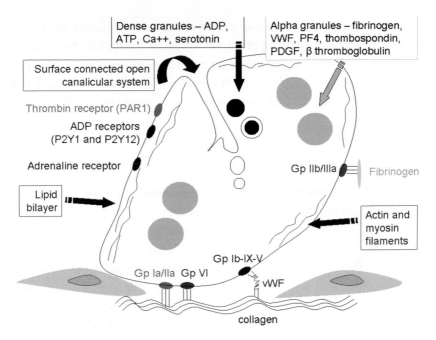

Fig. 11.3. A diagram of a platelet showing some of the components that are crucial for function. The platelet is enclosed by a lipid bilayer membrane, which when altered by platelet activation, provides phospholipid to interact with factors IXa, VIIIa and Ca^{++} and also with factors Xa, Va and Ca^{++}. The membrane lipid is also the source of arachidonic acid, which is converted by cyclo-oxygenase to thromboxane A2, a potent aggregant. Embedded in the membrane are various receptors: a thrombin receptor; several types of receptor for adenosine diphosphate (ADP); an adrenaline receptor; platelet glycoprotein (Gp) IIb/IIIa which, when its conformation is altered, is able to bind fibrinogen; GpIa/IIa and Gp VI, both of which can bind to exposed collagen; and Gp Ib-IX-V, which can bind to von Willebrand factor (VWF) and thus to collagen. Activated platelets are bound to each other by fibrinogen molecules, which bind to altered Gp IIb/IIIa on adjacent platelets. The platelet has various types of granules among which are the dense bodies (containing ADP, adenosine triphosphate [ATP], serotonin [a vasoconstrictor] and Ca^{++}) and the α granules (containing fibrinogen, fibronectin, VWF, platelet factor 4 [PF4, a heparin antagonist], thrombospondin, platelet-derived growth factor [PDGF] and β thromboglobulin). When platelets are activated, granule contents are discharged into the surface-connected canalicular system and are thus able to activate other platelets. Both thromboxane A2 and ADP enhance platelet aggregation induced by weak aggregants. Platelet shape is maintained by actin and myosin filaments, which are responsible for platelet contraction after activation.

The assembly of enzyme-cofactor-substrate complexes by binding to negatively charged phospholipid surfaces provided by activated platelets is an important element of the coagulation pathway. Activation of the platelets is also completed by the action of thrombin and so the primary and secondary coagulation mechanisms function together and are interdependent.

The vessel wall and haemostasis

The primary function of the vessel wall in health is to prevent thrombosis and to maintain the flow of blood. This is achieved by the surface expression of molecules with anticoagulant function such as tissue factor pathway inhibitor, thrombomodulin, heparans and the endothelial protein C receptor. The endothelium also actively releases prostacyclin and nitric oxide (NO), which inhibit platelet activation. These processes can be downregulated in response to inflammation or injury. In response to damage, a vasoconstrictor response will also act to reduce blood loss.

In Vitro Coagulation

Blood that is shed from the body forms a clot. Coagulation is initiated by contact with various negatively charged surfaces including glass. This route, via what is called 'contact activation,' is known as the 'intrinsic pathway' because it appears to be an intrinsic property of the blood. The contact pathway utilises factor XII (and also prekallikrein and high molecular weight kininogen) but is not an important route for coagulation *in vivo* and deficiencies of these factors do not result in an increased tendency to bleeding.

Understanding laboratory tests of coagulation requires knowledge of the intrinsic pathway and an extrinsic pathway as they operate *in vitro* (Fig. 11.4). This is somewhat different from the complex interactions that occur *in vivo*. The two pathways share a final common pathway.

Limitation of Coagulation and Fibrinolysis

Flowing blood does not clot in normal blood vessels since endothelial cells provide a barrier between the blood and procoagulant extracellular

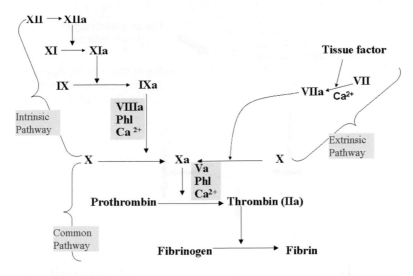

Fig. 11.4. Blood coagulation *in vitro*. The intrinsic and extrinsic systems are conceived as separate entities. It will be seen that, *in vitro*, factor XII has a significant role in contact activation and the intrinsic pathway.

proteins, such as collagen. In addition, endothelial cells secrete NO and prostacyclin. Both of these dilate vessels and prostacyclin also inhibits platelet adhesion. Endothelial cells also express thrombomodulin, which helps to limit coagulation. Normally, coagulation occurs only at the site of injury, since that is where tissue factor is activated and where platelets are exposed to subendothelial matrix; the platelet aggregates that form at that site tether the developing clot and help to limit it to that site.

The coagulation cascade leads to rapid generation of procoagulant proteins so that haemostasis is achieved and blood loss is limited. However, if this process were not limited, extensive unwanted thrombosis would ensue. Uncontrolled thrombin generation would convert the circulating blood into a giant blood clot. Coagulation is normally localised to the site of injury and is controlled by a number of naturally occurring anticoagulant proteins, which are activated during haemostasis. These anticoagulants include protein S, protein C and antithrombin, and will be discussed in Chapter 12.

Once haemostasis has been achieved it is desirable for the blood clot to be lysed so that blood flow is restored to the previously damaged

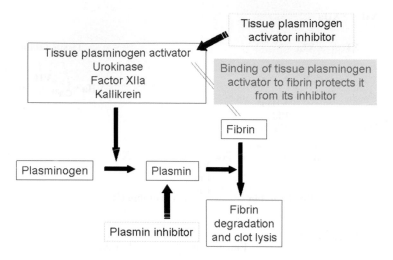

Fig. 11.5.   A diagram of fibrinolysis. Inhibitors are shown in red.

tissue. This is achieved by a process known as fibrinolysis. Fibrinolysis is initiated by the formation of the fibrin clot itself. Formation of fibrin exposes binding sites for tissue plasminogen activator and plasminogen which are normally both present in plasma but are now brought into close proximity. This greatly facilitates the conversion of plasminogen into the active fibrinolytic enzyme, plasmin, by tissue plasminogen activator (Fig. 11.5). Thus plasmin generation is usually limited to the region of the clot and if plasmin diffuses into plasma it is inactivated by the circulating plasmin inhibitor (previously known as α_2 antiplasmin). Plasmin cleaves fibrin to form fibrin degradation products (among which is D-dimer). There are also other physiological activators of plasminogen but these are probably more important in extravascular tissues (Fig. 11.5).

Assessment of Coagulation Status

Assessment of coagulation status requires both a clinical assessment and laboratory tests. Depending on the clinical features, it may be necessary to assess both the adequacy of coagulation factors and platelet number and function.

Clinical assessment of coagulation

Clinical assessment includes a personal and family history, a drug history and a physical examination. The clinical history includes that of the presenting complaint and of previous bleeding episodes, also taking note of the patient's response to previous haemostatic challenge. A history of dental interventions and minor as well as major surgery should be sought. Mothers of children should be asked if there was bleeding from the umbilical cord or following circumcision of male infants. If there has been previous haemorrhage, the nature and severity must be assessed. It is diagnostically important to know if bleeding is characteristic of a platelet defect or of a coagulation factor deficiency (Box 11.1). Severity of haemorrhage can be established by an assessment of duration of bleeding, how much blood was lost and whether hospitalisation or blood transfusion was required. Family history should include not only parents and siblings but also male maternal relatives since some congenital coagulation factor deficiencies have an X-linked recessive inheritance. Drug history should include establishing if the patient is taking aspirin or nonsteroidal anti-inflammatory agents, which interfere with platelet function.

Box 11.1
Differences between bleeding due to platelet defects
and due to coagulation factor deficiency

Bleeding due to thrombocytopenia or platelet functional defects is mainly into the skin and mucous membranes (epistaxis, bleeding gums, menorrhagia) and occurs immediately following injury
Bleeding due to a coagulation factor deficiency is mainly into deep tissues such as muscles and joints, and may be delayed

---

Physical examination should look for evidence of haemorrhage, including the presence of petechiae, ecchymoses or bruises (see Table 11.1), bleeding from venipuncture sites and also evidence of any systemic disease that could cause abnormal haemostasis, e.g. liver or renal disease. Evidence should be sought of any inherited or acquired blood

Table 11.1.   Some terminology used in coagulation.

Term	Meaning
Purpura	Bleeding into the skin and mucous membranes (can be thrombocytopenic or non-thrombocytopenic)
Petechia (plural petechiae)	Pinpoint cutaneous haemorrhages, a form of purpura
Ecchymosis (plural ecchymoses)	Large cutaneous haemorrhages, a form of purpura
Bruise	Bleeding into subcutaneous tissues

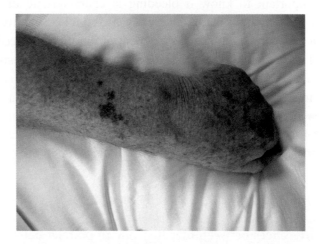

Fig. 11.6.   'Senile purpura' on the arm of an elderly man. This type of purpura occurs particularly on the hands and arms and is due to atrophy of soft tissues with ageing.

vessel or connective tissue abnormality that could cause haemorrhage, such as 'senile purpura' (Fig. 11.6), scurvy (perifollicular haemorrhage and corkscrew hairs), abnormally large or delicate scars, hereditary haemorrhagic telangiectasia (telangiectasia on lips or tongue) or Ehlers–Danlos syndrome.

Laboratory assessment of coagulation

A 'coagulation screen' always includes a prothrombin time and an activated partial thromboplastin time. It may also include a thrombin time and

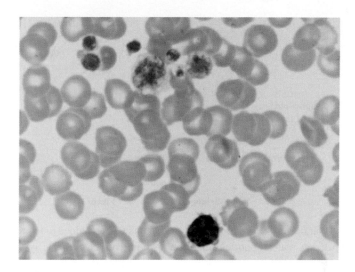

Fig. 11.7. Blood film of one of two sisters with autosomal recessive thrombocytopenia with giant platelets and impaired platelet function (suspected Bernard–Soulier syndrome).

an assay of fibrinogen. Coagulation tests are usually performed on platelet-poor plasma, i.e. plasma from blood that has been anticoagulated with sodium citrate and has been centrifuged to remove platelets. A platelet count should be performed and a blood film should be examined since some congenital defects of platelet function are associated with large platelets or poorly granulated platelets (Fig. 11.7). It is important to note that the 'coagulation screen' tests only a very small portion of the entire haemostatic mechanism and even this with limited sensitivity. In the presence of a suggestive clinical history, individual coagulation factors and platelet function may require specific assessment.

The prothrombin time

The prothrombin time (PT) assesses the extrinsic pathway (Fig. 11.8). A 'complete thromboplastin' containing tissue factor and phospholipid is added as well as calcium to reverse the effect of the citrate anticoagulant. The time until the appearance of a clot is then measured and is usually of the order of 12–14 seconds. The test is dependent on factors VII, X, V and II (prothrombin).

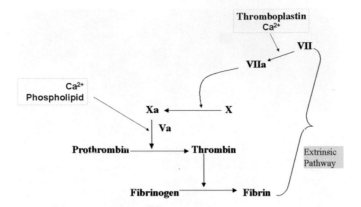

Fig.11.8. A diagram of the prothrombin time. Factors that are added to the test tube containing the patient's platelet-poor plasma are shown in red. The extrinsic system is tested.

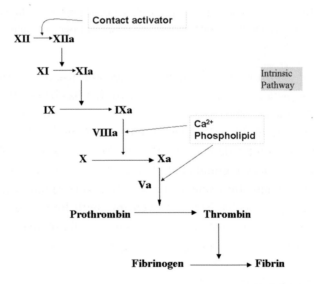

Fig. 11.9. A diagram of the activated partial thromboplastin time. Factors that are added to the test tube containing the patient's platelet-poor plasma are shown in red. The intrinsic system is tested.

The activated partial thromboplastin time

The activated partial thromboplastin time (APTT) assesses the intrinsic pathway (Figure 11.9). A contact activator is added, together with calcium and a 'partial thromboplastin.' A partial thromboplastin does not activate the extrinsic pathway but replaces platelet phospholipid in the steps where it is required in the intrinsic and common pathway. The test is dependent on factors XII, XI, IX, VIII, X, V and II. The normal range is usually of the order of 30–40 seconds but varies considerably according to the specific reagents used.

The thrombin time

In the thrombin time (TT), thrombin is added to plasma and the time taken for clotting to occur is recorded. A normal result is dependent on the presence of an adequate amount of normally functioning fibrinogen and on the absence of factors that might inhibit conversion of fibrinogen to fibrin, such as exogenous heparin or endogenous fibrin degradation products. The concentration of thrombin added to the plasma sample is adjusted so that clotting usually occurs in 15–20 seconds.

Fibrinogen assay

The thrombin time will detect only a severe deficiency of fibrinogen. It can be useful to measure the actual quantity present using a functional or immunological assay. The normal concentration is about 1.8–3.6 g/l.

Platelet function tests

Platelet function has traditionally been tested by a bleeding time or platelet aggregation studies. A bleeding time is performed by inflating a blood pressure cuff and making a standardised puncture or incision of the forearm; the duration of bleeding is then recorded. The bleeding time is about 2–6 minutes from a puncture and somewhat longer from an incision. The test is now rarely performed because it is poorly reproducible, operator-dependent and a poor predictor of bleeding problems. To some extent the bleeding time has been replaced by newer methods of testing platelet function such as the PFA-100 instrument that aspirates a blood sample through a capillary into a cartridge that contains either collagen plus adrenaline or collagen plus ADP. The time for occlusion of the aperture by a platelet thrombus is recorded. This test requires normal platelet number and function as well as VWF but will not detect some milder forms of platelet defect. In platelet aggregation studies, various platelet aggregants, such as adrenaline, ADP, collagen or ristocetin, are added to platelet-rich plasma; the rate and completeness of platelet aggregation are studied by recording changes in optical density

Other coagulation tests

Each individual coagulation factor can be assayed. The principle of these tests is an assessment of the ability of the test plasma to correct the clotting defect in plasma that is deficient in only a single factor.

Inherited Coagulation Defects

All inherited defects of coagulation are uncommon or rare. Von Willebrand disease may have a prevalence as high as 1% but many cases are mild or even asymptomatic. All other disorders are rare or very rare. Haemophilia A (factor VIII deficiency) has a birth incidence in males of about one in 5000. Factor IX deficiency, also referred to as haemophilia B, is about a quarter as common as haemophilia A. All other inherited coagulation defects are very rare, with the exception of factor XI deficiency among Ashkenazi Jews.

Haemophilia A

Haemophilia A, also referred to simply as haemophilia, results from an X-linked inherited deficiency of factor VIII. Some cases are due to spontaneous mutations in the factor VIII gene so not all patients have a positive family history. Factor VIII concentration may be less than 1%, leading to a very severe bleeding disorder (Fig. 11.10). There is spontaneous haemorrhage into joints and muscles, disproportionate bleeding following minor trauma or surgery and sometimes, gastrointestinal haemorrhage, haematuria or intracranial haemorrhage. The PT and TT are normal whereas the APTT is prolonged (study Figs. 11.4, 11.8 and 11.9 to understand why). Confirmation is by assay of factor VIII. There is

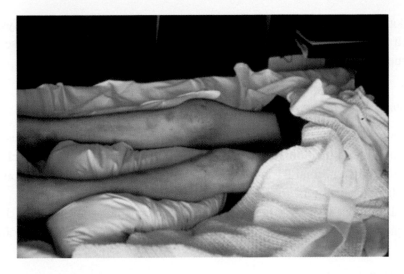

Fig. 11.10. Bilateral knee haemarthroses in haemophilia. There are also some bruises.

reduction of factor VIII clotting activity whereas the carrier molecule, VWF, is normal.

Haemophilia A is ideally treated with recombinant human factor VIII. Alternatively, in countries that cannot afford this product, treatment can be with plasma-derived factor VIII concentrate or with cryoprecipitate, a blood product prepared by freezing and thawing plasma and isolating the cryoprecipitate, which is slowest to redissolve. Cryoprecipitate contains fibrinogen as well as factor VIII so can also be used for other purposes. Ideally, parents and children should learn injection techniques since home treatment avoids any delay in treatment and thus lessens morbidity. The half-life of factor VIII is short (about 12 hours) but nevertheless it is possible to give prophylactic factor VIII alternate days or three times weekly to children with severe haemophilia in order to prevent haemorrhage and thus avoid chronic joint and other tissue damage; the incidence of cerebral haemorrhage is also reduced by prophylaxis. Some 10–15% of patients with severe haemophilia develop antibodies that act as inhibitors of factor VIII; alternative forms of treatment are then needed. Patients with mild haemophilia can be treated with desmopressin, which leads to release of VWF and factor VIII from endothelial cells; it is often given together with an inhibitor of fibrinolysis, such as tranexamic acid, since its administration also leads to release of tissue plasminogen activator.

Haemophilia B

Haemophilia B or factor IX deficiency has similar clinical features to haemophilia A including an X-linked recessive inheritance. It is also characterised by a normal PT and TT and a prolonged APTT. Confirmation of the diagnosis is by factor IX assay.

Treatment is with a factor IX concentrate, which can be given less frequently than factor VIII because its half-life is approximately 24 hours.

Von Willebrand disease

Von Willebrand disease is an inherited deficiency of VWF or VWF activity. VWF is synthesised in megakaryocytes and endothelial cells although only the endothelium contributes to the levels measured in plasma. Deficiency of VWF, particularly if severe, can also result in deficiency of factor VIII since VWF transports and stabilises factor VIII. Most cases show an autosomal dominant inheritance with the severity of disease varying greatly between families. Occasional severe cases have autosomal recessive inheritance. Since VWF is required for normal platelet function, patients with VWF have bleeding from mucosal surfaces as well as deep-seated bleeding in those cases with low levels of factor VIII. The coagulation screen is frequently normal but the APTT may be prolonged if the factor VIII is low. The bleeding time is prolonged in severe cases but often normal in milder forms of the disease. VWF activity in plasma can be measured by the ability of the plasma to induce platelet agglutination in the presence of the antibiotic ristocetin; this is called ristocetin cofactor activity.

Treatment can be with intermediate purity factor VIII concentrate, which contains VWF as well as factor VIII or with high-purity VWF concentrate. It is also possible to treat mild cases with tranexamic acid (to inhibit fibrinolysis) or with desmopressin.

Table 11.2. Laboratory tests results in inherited defects of coagulation factors.

Deficient factor	APTT	PT	TT
XII*	Prolonged	Normal	Normal
XI	Prolonged	Normal	Normal
IX	Prolonged	Normal	Normal
VIII	Prolonged	Normal	Normal
X	Prolonged	Prolonged	Normal
V	Prolonged	Prolonged	Normal
II (prothrombin)	Prolonged	Prolonged	Normal
I (hypofibrinogenaemia)	Prolonged	Prolonged	Prolonged
I (dysfibrinogenaemia)	Prolonged	Prolonged	Prolonged
VII	Normal	Prolonged	Normal
XIII†	Normal	Normal	Normal

* No clinical coagulation defect present.
† Alternative test assessing stability of clot is needed.

Other inherited coagulation factor deficiencies

Table 11.2 summarises the test results expected in other inherited defects of coagulation factors. These deficiencies are all rare but the table illustrates how coagulation tests can be interpreted.

Acquired Defects of Coagulation

Acquired defects of coagulation can result from: (i) defective synthesis or increased utilisation of coagulation factors; (ii) dilution following transfusion for massive haemorrhage; (iii) the development of a coagulation factor inhibitor; or (iv) the presence of a drug, such as heparin, that inhibits coagulation. The two common causes of defective synthesis are liver disease and administration of vitamin K antagonists for the prevention of thromboembolic disease.

Vitamin K deficiency or antagonism

The commonly used oral anticoagulants are vitamin K antagonists, which by blocking the recycling of vitamin K reduce the ability to perform the final step (γ-carboxylation) in the synthesis of factors II, VII, IX and X. Deficiency of these factors interferes with both the intrinsic (factor IX), extrinsic (factor VII) and common (factors X and II) pathways. As would be expected, both the PT and APPT are abnormal but in practice the PT is relatively more prolonged. The TT is normal. A similar coagulation abnormality can be seen in obstructive jaundice, when there is poor absorption of the fat-soluble vitamins including vitamin K. Coeliac disease can also lead to a bleeding disorder due to malabsorption of vitamin K. Neonates are prone to vitamin K deficiency in the first week of life but in most countries this is prevented by administration of vitamin K.

Bleeding resulting from deficiency of vitamin K is readily treated by parenteral administration of the vitamin. However, correction of the defect may take 24 hours or longer and so if rapid correction is needed the missing factors are replaced using concentrate or, if this is not available, fresh-frozen plasma.

Liver disease

Since all coagulation factors except VWF are synthesised in the liver, severe liver disease will cause a prolongation of the PT and APTT. In severe liver disease a reduced fibrinogen concentration may be encountered. Some forms of liver disease, particularly carcinoma, are associated with an acquired dysfibrinogenaemia characterised by prolongation of the TT and elevation of the fibrinogen concentration. This is not associated with an increase in bleeding. If there is an obstructive element to the liver disease, specific deficiency of vitamin-dependent factors occurs in addition to the generalised reduced rate of synthesis of all factors. There is impaired clearance of activated coagulation factors (making disseminated intravascular coagulation more likely) and of tissue plasminogen activator (leading to enhanced fibrinolysis). Thrombocytopenia as a result of hypersplenism can also be present.

Renal disease

Renal failure can lead to haemorrhage as a result of inhibition of platelet function.

Massive transfusion

During blood loss, replacement is initially with reconstituted plasma-reduced red cells and colloid solutions. If it is clear that blood loss is going to be very considerable, replacement should also include fresh-frozen plasma and platelet concentrates. If replacement does not keep pace with loss, a global defect of clotting will occur, characterised by prolongation of the PT, APPT and TT, a reduced fibrinogen concentration and a low platelet count. The coagulation defect may be aggravated by disseminated intravascular coagulation, e.g. triggered by trauma, acidosis and hypoxia, and by activation of fibrinolysis. Once a serious clotting defect has developed, management is with transfusion of fresh-frozen plasma (which contains all clotting factors), cryoprecipitate (supplying factor VIII, factor XIII and fibrinogen) and platelet concentrates.

Disseminated intravascular coagulation

Disseminated intravascular coagulation (DIC) is a haemorrhagic disorder with disseminated activation of coagulation within the circulation accompanied, when the process is acute, by increased fibrinolysis. Some of the causes are shown in Table 11.3. Clinical features are haemorrhage, including diffuse oozing from venipuncture sites and from small vessels in surgical wounds or at sites of trauma. There is also end-organ impairment, related to intravascular fibrin deposition, affecting lungs, kidneys and brain. Increased utilisation of coagulation factors leads to a global

Table 11.3.   **Some causes of disseminated intravascular coagulation.**

Cause	Examples
Infection	Meningococcal septicaemia, other septicaemia
Tissue injury related to trauma, shock, hypoxia and acidosis	Trauma, hypotension due to acute blood loss including that due to injury and obstetric misadventures, burns
Release of procoagulant substances into the circulation	Acute promyelocytic leukaemia, concealed antepartum haemorrhage, amniotic fluid embolism, disseminated carcinoma, incompatible blood transfusion

coagulation defect with prolongation of PT, APTT and TT, fibrinogen deficiency, presence of fibrin degradation products and thrombocytopenia. Sometimes the blood becomes incoagulable. The prolongation of the TT is due not only to fibrinogen deficiency but also to inhibition of the conversion of fibrinogen to fibrin by the anticoagulant action of fibrin degradation products. Haemorrhage may be aggravated by abnormal platelet function, e.g. if the patient has been on cardiopulmonary bypass or has been taking aspirin or other anti-platelet drugs or if there is renal failure. Tests indicated in suspected DIC are PT, APTT, TT, fibrinogen assay, measurement of fibrin degradation products and a full blood count including a platelet count. A commonly used test for fibrin degradation products is a measurement of D-dimer, this breakdown product of fibrin being formed only when there has been cross-linking of fibrin and subsequent fibrinolysis.

Management is by transfusion of red cells, platelets, fresh-frozen plasma and cryoprecipitate. Vigorous efforts to correct the underlying cause as well as supportive care to try to correct hypotension, hypoxia and acidosis are also of considerable importance.

Coagulation inhibitors

Some coagulation inhibitors lead to destruction of coagulation factors and serious bleeding. Others interfere with coagulation tests without causing bleeding. The clinical significance clearly differs.

Coagulation inhibitors that can lead to bleeding

Coagulation inhibitors that can aggravate bleeding or lead to bleeding can develop not only in patients with an inherited deficiency of a coagulation factor but also in previously healthy people, occurring as an autoimmune phenomenon. Sometimes their occurrence is related to pregnancy or exposure to a drug (e.g. penicillin) or is associated with a known autoimmune disease (e.g. rheumatoid arthritis). Inhibitors directed at factor VIII are the most common. Coagulation tests are similar to those found in deficiency of a coagulation factor but with the difference that, in a deficiency, mixing of normal plasma with the patient's plasma corrects the defect whereas in the presence of an inhibitor it does not. Treatment can be with high doses of the relevant coagulant factor or with coagulation factors designed to bypass the defect (e.g. in the case of a factor VIII inhibitor, porcine factor VIII, prothrombin complex or activated prothrombin complex [contain factors II, IX and X and possibly VII], or recombinant factor VIIa). In the longer term, immunosuppressive therapy may be useful. Management is difficult and there is significant mortality.

Lupus anticoagulant

This *in vitro* coagulation inhibitor develops both in patients with systemic lupus erythematosus and as a primary autoimmune disease. It is an antiphospholipid antibody that interferes with coagulation tests that require a phospholipid, particularly the APTT and is further discussed on page 249.

Thrombocytopenia

Thrombocytopenia may be inherited or acquired. Inherited thrombocytopenia is rare. There may be associated giant platelets or platelet dysfunction. Acquired thrombocytopenia is common. Some of the causes are shown in Table 11.4. Drug-induced thrombocytopenia is usually the

Table 11.4.   **Some causes of acquired thrombocytopenia.**

Mechanism	Examples
Decreased platelet production	Acute leukaemia, aplastic anaemia, administration of cytotoxic chemotherapy
Increased consumption	Disseminated intravascular coagulation, massive haemorrhage, thrombotic thrombocytopenic purpura
Increased destruction	Autoimmune thrombocytopenic purpura, alloimmune thrombocytopenia (e.g. in the fetus and neonate), drug-induced thrombocytopenia including heparin-induced thrombocytopenia, post-infection thrombocytopenia, autoimmune thrombocytopenia in HIV (human immunodeficiency virus) infection, post-transfusion purpura
Pooling in an enlarged spleen*	Hypersplenism, e.g. in portal cirrhosis

* Usually about one-third of the body's platelets are found in the spleen but in hypersplenism it may be up to 90%.

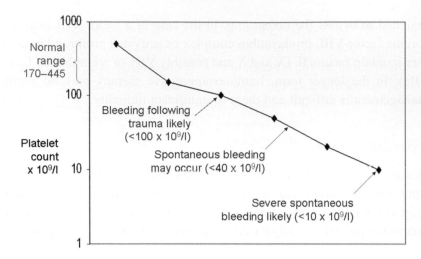

Fig. 11.11. A diagram of a falling platelet count showing the points at which significant haemorrhage may occur and is likely to occur.

result of an antibody that recognises a drug (or metabolite) bound to a specific platelet glycoprotein, usually either glycoprotein IIb/IIIa or Ib/IX. It is usually severe. Heparin-induced thrombocytopenia (see page 253) has different characteristics.

Haemorrhage due either to thrombocytopenia or to impaired platelet function can be treated by platelet transfusions. To some extent the probability of haemorrhage can be predicted from the platelet count (Fig. 11.11). In some clinical circumstance, e.g. in treating patients with acute leukaemia, prophylactic platelet transfusions are given when the platelet count is very low to prevent haemorrhage occurring; this is usually done when the platelet count falls below $10–15 \times 10^9/l$. Associated inflammation will increase the tendency to bleed at any given platelet count.

Autoimmune thrombocytopenic purpura

Autoimmune thrombocytopenic purpura, previously known as idiopathic thrombocytopenic purpura (ITP), results from production of an auto-antibody directed at platelet antigens. Splenic and other macrophages have receptors for the Fc fragment of immunoglobulin G and bind and phagocytose the platelet. ITP can occur as an isolated phenomenon or as one feature of an autoimmune disease. It can also occur as a complication of chronic lymphocytic leukaemia or lymphoma. Occasionally, it coexists with autoimmune haemolytic anaemia (Evans' syndrome) or neutropenia. Immune thrombocytopenia also occurs with an increased incidence when there is infection by the hepatitis C virus, the human immunodeficiency virus (HIV) or *Helicobacter pylori*.

ITP appears to be a somewhat different condition in children and adults. In children the peak incidence is around 5 years of age and frequency is the same in boys and girls. It often remits spontaneously, it is suspected that it is triggered by an infection and treatment is usually not needed. In adults, peak incidence is in young adults and it is more common in women than in men; it is more likely to become chronic and treatment is usually needed.

Clinical features

Presentation is usually with bruising or with epistaxis or other bleeding from mucosal surfaces. Cerebral haemorrhage is an uncommon complication. Physical examination shows purpura (petechiae and ecchymoses) and bruises (Fig. 11.12). There may be blood blisters in the mouth. When ITP is a feature of an autoimmune disease, such as systemic lupus erythematosus or rheumatoid arthritis, there will be clinical features of the primary disease.

Laboratory features

The blood count and blood film confirm thrombocytopenia. If the condition is acute, the platelets are of normal size but if it is chronic there are some large platelets, which are haemostatically more effective.

Diagnosis and differential diagnosis

The blood count and film are important for the exclusion of other causes of thrombocytopenia, such as thrombotic thrombocytopenic purpura (see page 241) and acute leukaemia. A coagulation screen is always performed,

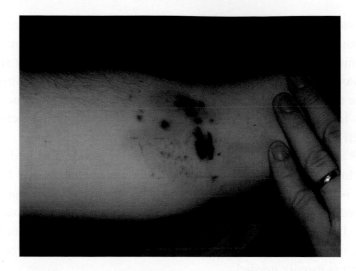

Fig. 11.12. The arm of a young man with autoimmune thrombocytopenic purpura showing petechiae and bleeding at venipuncture sites.

in order to exclude DIC as an alternative cause of thrombocytopenia. The coagulation screen may also give evidence of a lupus anticoagulant. Autoantibodies are tested for, including antinuclear factor, anti-DNA antibodies and anticardiolipin antibodies. However, testing for platelet autoantibodies is not useful because of poor sensitivity and specificity of available tests. In adults, a bone marrow aspirate is usually performed and shows that megakaryocyte numbers are usually normal or increased. In children, this investigation can usually be avoided as the clinical picture is very typical; however, if treatment with corticosteroids is considered to be indicated then it may be performed (because of anxiety that thrombocytopenia may be the result of an otherwise unsuspected acute lymphoblastic leukaemia).

Management

Platelet transfusion is indicated only if there is life-threatening haemorrhage, since the presence of an antiplatelet antibody means that transfused platelets survive only briefly in the circulation. Children are usually not actively treated. In adults, the immune process is treated initially with corticosteroids. High-dose intravenous immunoglobulin or anti-D immunoglobulin (for Rh D-positive patients) can be given if rapid elevation of the platelet counts is required but their use does not affect the underlying disease. The aim of treatment is to prevent bleeding, rather than to raise the platelet count to normal; a platelet count of 20–$50 \times 10^9/l$ may well be adequate. If the disease proves to be refractory, other options include other immunosuppressive drugs, splenectomy (with appropriate prophylaxis against infection) and agents that mimic the action of thrombopoietin and increase platelet production. Aspirin and other drugs that either interfere with platelet function or increase the risk of gastrointestinal haemorrhage should be avoided.

Thrombotic thrombocytopenic purpura

Thrombotic thrombocytopenic purpura results from platelet aggregation in small vessels and is characterised by a pentad of clinical and laboratory features — fever, neurological abnormalities, thrombocytopenia, microangiopathic haemolytic anaemia and renal impairment. It results from a deficiency of VWF-cleaving protease (ADAMTS13), usually as a result of production of an autoantibody directed at this factor but inherited forms are also seen. As a result, ultra-large molecules of VWF are present, which bind spontaneously to platelets trapping them on the endothelial surface. The platelet microthrombi cause the microangiopathic haemolytic anaemia. This condition is rare but its diagnosis is nevertheless important since urgent treatment is needed.

Clinical features

Presentation is usually with symptoms of anaemia, purpura, neurological impairment and fever.

Laboratory features

The blood count and film confirm thrombocytopenia and in addition show red cell fragments and polychromasia. Serum creatinine is elevated and there is biochemical evidence of haemolysis.

Diagnosis and differential diagnosis

Diagnosis is based on the presence of all or most of the characteristic pentad of clinical and laboratory features. The differential diagnosis includes other causes of thrombocytopenia and of red cell fragmentation.

Management

Treatment is by plasmapheresis to remove the autoantibody and replace the ADAMTS13, often followed by immunosuppressive treatment. Platelet transfusion is contraindicated since it may aggravate the microangiopathy and organ damage.

Defective Platelet Function

Defective platelet function may be inherited or acquired.

Inherited defects of platelet function

Inherited defects of platelet function are rare. There is sometimes associated thrombocytopenia. Platelet size may be increased or there may be hypogranularity of platelets. Diagnosis is by blood count and film, and platelet aggregation studies. Deficiency of platelet glycoprotein can be assessed most readily by flow cytometry and platelet granule content by measurement of platelet nucleotides (ADP and adenosine triphosphate [ATP]). Management is by platelet transfusion if serious haemorrhage occurs or prophylactically if there is an urgent need for surgery. Mild defects may also respond to desmopressin.

Acquired defects of platelet function

The most common cause of acquired platelet dysfunction is exposure to drugs that interfere with platelet function. As well as aspirin, many patients are prescribed dipyridamole or inhibitors of the ADP receptor such as clopidogrel to therapeutically reduce platelet function. Platelet inhibition also results from nonsteroidal anti-inflammatory drugs prescribed for other indications; these drugs can also be bought over the counter. In the myelodysplastic syndromes and acute myeloid leukaemia, platelets may be intrinsically abnormal. Impaired function due to accumulation of guanidinosuccinic acid is common in renal failure. Platelet dysfunction due to prior activation and granule release occurs following cardiopulmonary bypass and in DIC. In essential thrombocythaemia with very high counts, there may be paradoxical bleeding because of acquired von Willebrand disease, which leads to platelet dysfunction (see page 191).

Management of acquired defects of platelet function is by control of the primary condition, withdrawal of relevant drugs (if possible) and, if serious haemorrhage occurs, platelet transfusion. Following cardiopulmonary bypass and in DIC and myeloid neoplasms, platelet transfusions are indicated not only when the platelet count is low but also when there is bleeding at a platelet count that would normally be adequate for haemostasis.

Conclusions

Clinical history is the most important means of detecting abnormal coagulation or platelet function and often suggests whether any defect is in coagulation factors or in platelets. A full blood count and film and a coagulation screen is indicated when clinical history suggest a possible defect. These basic investigations are supplemented by other tests when clinically indicated.

Test Case 11.1

A 57-year-old previously healthy woman presents with the gradual onset of painless jaundice. Carcinoma of the pancreas is suspected and she has an FBC and coagulation screen performed prior to planned endoscopy. The FBC is normal but the coagulation screen shows:

Prothrombin time 25 sec (normal range [NR] 12–14)

Activated partial thromboplastin time 45 sec (NR 30–40)

Thrombin time 20 sec (control 21 sec)

Fibrinogen 4.5 g/l (NR 1.8–3.6)

Questions

1. What is the most likely cause of the coagulation factor deficiency?
2. Which coagulation factors are likely to be deficient?
3. Why if the fibrinogen concentration increased?

Write down your answers before checking the correct answer (page 327) and re-reading any relevant part of the chapter.

Test Case 11.2

A 27-year-old previously healthy woman presents with a haematemesis. She has not suffered any indigestion and has not been taking aspirin or any other antiplatelet drugs. While an urgent gastroscopy is being arranged, the house surgeon takes a full history and finds that she has suffered from recurrent nose bleeds and has always had heavy periods. She is aware that her mother also suffered from nose bleeds. A coagulation screen and subsequent assays shows:

Prothrombin time 13 sec (normal range [NR] 12–14)
Activated partial thromboplastin time 55 sec (NR 30–40)
Thrombin time 19 sec (control 21 sec)
Factor VIII 25% (NR 50–150)
Von Willebrand factor 17 % (NR 50–200)

Questions

1. What is the most likely cause of the bleeding disorder?
2. What would you expect a bleeding time to show and why?
3. Why is the factor VIII low?

Write down your answers before checking the correct answer (page 327) and re-reading any relevant part of the chapter.

12

Thrombosis and Its Management — Anticoagulant, Antiplatelet and Thrombolytic Therapy

What Do You Have to Know?

☞ Why thrombosis occurs and how it can be prevented
☞ The nature of thrombophilia and how it is managed
☞ The clinical role and management of heparin therapy
☞ The clinical role and management of oral anticoagulants
☞ The role of antiplatelet drugs
☞ The role of thrombolytic therapy

Haemostasis and Thrombosis

Haemostasis is essential to prevent fatal blood loss following injury. Normally, coagulation is limited to the site of injury. Generation of clot is also controlled by the action of a number of naturally occurring anticoagulants, including antithrombin, tissue factor pathway inhibitor (TFPI) and activated protein C, which are activated whenever blood coagulation occurs. Both protein C and protein S are vitamin K-dependent serine proteases. Protein C is activated by thrombin complexed to endothelial membrane thrombomodulin (Fig. 12.1). In turn, protein C, with protein S

245

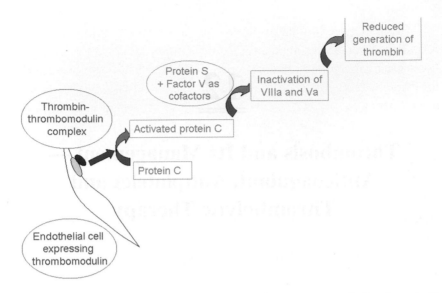

Fig. 12.1.   The interaction of naturally occurring anticoagulants, protein S and protein C.

and factor V as cofactors, inactivates the activated forms of factor V and factor VIII, thus serving to control thrombin generation.

Perturbation of this physiological response to injury can lead to a pathological process known as thrombosis, in which clotting occurs in arteries, arterioles, capillaries, venules or veins, leading to disability or death.

In developed societies, atherosclerosis and arterial thrombosis are responsible for significant morbidity and mortality. As unhealthy diets, lack of exercise and obesity are becoming common also in developing countries this is becoming a global problem. A thrombus can narrow or totally block a coronary vessel, leading to myocardial ischaemia or infarction. Thrombosis in cerebral blood vessels can lead to infarction of part of the brain, recognised clinically as a 'stroke'. Ischaemic (as opposed to haemorrhagic) stroke can also result from embolism of a blood clot to the brain. A frequent underlying cause of this is atrial fibrillation, which is common in an ageing population. The ineffective contractions of the atrium lead to formation of blood clots in the atrial appendage; these can embolise from the left atrium to the brain.

A further large burden of disease and a significant number of deaths results from venous thrombosis and pulmonary embolism. Venous thrombosis usually occurs in the deep veins of the legs and pelvis with part of the thrombus sometimes breaking free and embolising to the lung. Venous thromboembolism (VTE) is a common condition with an overall incidence of 1–3 per 1000 per year. In developed countries it accounts for 5–10% of deaths of hospitalised patients and 20–30% of deaths related to pregnancy and childbirth. In the UK it is a leading cause of maternal death.

Morbidity and mortality can also result from deposition of fibrin and aggregation of platelets within capillaries, leading to end organ damage and thrombocytopenia.

Anticoagulant and antiplatelet therapy has been developed in an attempt to deal with the disease burden resulting from thrombosis.

Aetiology of thrombosis

Thrombosis in arteries is usually the result of atheroma, which is predisposed to by hypertension, diabetes mellitus, hyperlipidaemia (including that related to obesity) and cigarette smoking. Atheroma leads to aggregation of platelets on the atheromatous plaque and subsequent thrombosis. Increased concentration of certain of the coagulation factors can predispose to arterial occlusion as can an increased platelet count and increased blood viscosity due to a high haematocrit. Polycythaemia vera and essential thrombocythaemia can thus predispose to arterial thrombosis.

Venous thrombosis is related mainly to an increased concentration of coagulation factors, to endothelial damage and to stasis within vessels including that due to partial obstruction by external pressure (as in pregnancy). A reduction in naturally occurring anticoagulants can also contribute. The contributing factors can be summarised as Virchow's triad of hypercoagulability, stasis and endothelial injury or dysfunction, two or three of which may co-exist (Fig. 12.2). There are many factors that increase the risk of venous thromboembolism, including pregnancy, childbirth, surgery, trauma, immobility (including long-distance travel), cancer, advancing age, a high haematocrit, oral contraceptives, hormone replacement therapy and administration of thalidomide or lenalidomide.

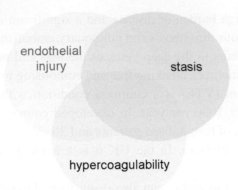

endothelial
injury

stasis

hypercoagulability

Fig. 12.2. A diagram illustrating Virchow's triad.

Thrombosis within the microcirculation can be the result of thrombocytosis, as in myeloproliferative neoplasms. It can also result from increased aggregability of platelets as a consequence of an increased concentration of ultra-large multimers of von Willebrand factor, as occurs in thrombotic thrombocytopenic purpura.

Management of thrombotic diseases requires not only pharmacological measures but also consideration of factors that contribute to atherosclerosis and increase the risk of thrombosis such as obesity, lack of exercise, hyperlipidaemia, hypertension, cigarette smoking and exposure to oral contraceptives or other hormones.

Thrombophilia

Some individuals have an increased tendency to VTE, related to inherited abnormalities of naturally occurring plasma proteins, either anticoagulant proteins or coagulation proteins. This is referred to as 'thrombophilia'. Some of these defects are uncommon but cause a marked increase in the risk of thrombosis. Others are very common but the degree of increase in risk is less. These inherited abnormalities are summarised in Table 12.1. Some patients who develop VTE benefit from investigation for thrombophilia since this information indicates the risk of further thrombosis and helps to determine the optimal length of anticoagulation. Such

Table 12.1. Inherited thrombophilia.

Defect	Prevalence in Caucasian populations	Increased risk of thrombosis in heterozygotes
Antithrombin deficiency[a]	1 in 2000	About 20-fold
Protein C deficiency[a]	3 in 1000	About 10-fold
Protein S deficiency[a]	1 in 700	About 8-fold
Factor V Leiden[b]	3–15%	About 3-fold
Factor II 20210G → A[b]	1–1.5%	About 5-fold

[a] Loss of function mutation in a gene for a naturally occurring anticoagulant.
[b] Gain of function in a coagulation factor gene.

investigation can reasonably be carried out in patients who are young (less than 55 years of age) or who have extensive thrombosis despite a trivial trigger or have pregnancy- or oestrogen-associated thrombosis or thrombosis in unusual sites.

Thrombophilia can also be the result of an acquired abnormality. The most important of these is the presence of the so-called 'lupus anticoagulant' (see below), an anticardiolipin antibody or both.

Inherited and acquired thrombophilic abnormalities are associated with an increased incidence of recurrent miscarriage and fetal loss. They can interact with other factors, such as surgery and immobility, that promote thrombosis in individuals who do not have thrombophilia.

Lupus anticoagulant

The lupus anticoagulant is an autoantibody, an antiphospholipid antibody, that inhibits coagulation in laboratory tests (hence its name) but in the patient actually predisposes to thrombosis. It can occur as one feature of systemic lupus erythematosus or can be an isolated phenomenon (primary antiphospholipid syndrome) characterised by both venous and arterial thromboses and pregnancy complications. There is an increased rate of recurrent miscarriage and fetal loss as a result of placental insufficiency. The lupus anticoagulant is an antiphospholipid antibody that interferes with phospholipid-dependent coagulation tests such as the activated partial thromboplastin time (APTT). There is often an associated anticardiolipin antibody.

Management is with oral anticoagulation therapy, for at least 6 months for VTE or lifelong when there is recurrent VTE or in arterial thrombosis. Low-dose aspirin plus low-dose heparin (usually low molecular weight heparin) is used for recurrent miscarriage.

The Need for Anticoagulant and Antiplatelet Therapy

The burden of vascular and venous thromboembolic disease has led to successful attempts to treat or prevent thrombosis by interfering with blood clotting or platelet action.

Anticoagulant therapy is also needed to prevent blood clotting during haemodialysis and heart-lung bypass and may be needed to maintain patency of arterial stents (e.g. in coronary arteries), arterial grafts for peripheral vascular disease or arteriovenous shunts (e.g. those established for haemodialysis).

The management of arterial and venous thrombosis may be achieved with a single agent but often requires the combination of more than one agent (see Table 12.4). Since therapy leads to an increased risk of haemorrhage, the use of such treatment requires a careful consideration of risks and benefits. Decisions on the choice of treatment should be evidence-based and appropriate to the specific clinical features of individual patients. Randomised trials and meta-analyses of similar trials provide a sound basis for treatment decisions.

The important anticoagulants that are well established in clinical use are heparin (used parenterally) and vitamin K antagonists (active orally). Newer agents include direct thrombin and direct anti-factor Xa inhibitors. The cost of newer agents is considerably higher than the costs of heparin and vitamin K antagonists, although there may be indirect savings if monitoring is not needed.

Non-Pharmacological Means of Reducing Venous Thromboembolism

Around one-quarter of all venous thromboembolism occurs in hospitalised patients. In surgical and high-risk medical patients the risk of thrombosis can be reduced by non-pharmacological means such as early ambulation, encouraging leg and foot exercises, graduated compression stockings and use of pneumatic compression devices. In pregnant women, avoiding unnecessary caesarean section reduces the incidence of venous thromboembolism.

Parenteral Anticoagulants

The most frequently used parenteral anticoagulant is heparin, either unfractionated or low molecular weight.

Heparin

Heparin is a heterogeneous mixture of sulphated polysaccharides. It is a naturally occurring anticoagulant that is found in human and animal tissues. As a therapeutic product it is extracted from animal tissues, e.g. pig intestines. Heparin can be either unfractionated heparin, with a mean molecular weight around 15 000 daltons, or low- molecular weight heparin, which has been depolymerised and has a molecular weight around 4000–5000 daltons. Heparin does not cross the placenta and is not secreted in breast milk. Hence it is the anticoagulant of choice in pregnancy.

Heparin has an anticoagulant effect when complexed in the circulation with antithrombin. The heparin-antithrombin complex inhibits factor XIa, factor IXa, factor Xa and thrombin (Fig. 12.3).

The main unwanted effect is haemorrhage. Less common is heparin-induced thrombocytopenia (see below). The long-term administration of heparin can lead to osteoporosis.

Unfractionated heparin

Unfractionated heparin can be administered intravenously, with a loading dose being followed by a continuous infusion, or can be given subcutaneously, twice daily. If given intravenously, the anticoagulant effect is immediate. The effect has largely disappeared by 6 hours from cessation of therapy but if necessary it can be reversed rapidly by the administration of protamine sulphate. Unfractionated heparin is indicated whenever urgent anticoagulation is required or in a clinically unstable

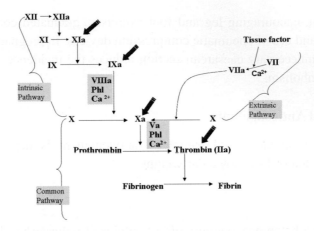

Fig. 12.3.   The sites of action of the heparin–antithrombin complex (red arrows). Note that an activated partial thromboplastin time will be affected by all four of these interactions.

patient in whom cessation or reversal of therapy may become necessary. It is used during cardiopulmonary bypass, being reversed at the end of the procedure by administration of protamine sulphate. It can be used during haemodialysis but low molecular weight heparin is an alternative. It is indicated in patients with acute coronary syndromes, in whom it reduces the risk of myocardial infarction and death. Heparin requires monitoring and dose adjustment based on the APTT.

Low molecular weight heparin

In comparison with unfractionated heparin, low molecular weight heparins, such as enoxaparin and tinziparin, have enhanced anti-Xa activity in relation to their anti-thrombin activity. They have a longer duration of action and can be administered subcutaneously once or twice daily. They do not usually require monitoring but, when monitoring is considered necessary, an anti-Xa assay can be used. Low molecular weight heparins are effective in venous thromboembolism prophylaxis and treatment and in acute coronary syndromes. They are less effectively neutralised by protamine sulphate than is unfractionated heparin.

Heparin-induced thrombocytopenia

In a minority of patients heparin, mainly unfractionated heparin, induces immune thrombocytopenia, usually between 5 and 10 days from the start of therapy. The mechanism is development of an antibody to the heparin–platelet factor 4 complex. The thrombocytopenia is not very severe (median platelet count at nadir $60 \times 10^9/l$) but is of considerable clinical importance because of an association with paradoxical arterial and venous thrombosis. It is managed by immediate cessation of heparin and replacement by another anticoagulant (see Table 12.4).

Other parenteral anticoagulants

Other parenteral anticoagulants are used is specific circumstances. They are summarised in Table 12.2.

Oral anticoagulant therapy

Traditional oral anticoagulants are vitamin K antagonists, although newer agents that directly inhibit thrombin or factor Xa are now available. They are summarised in Table 12.3.

Table 12.2. Parenteral anticoagulants.

Agent	Uses
Heparin (unfractionated or low molecular weight)	Prophylaxis and treatment of venous thromboembolism, myocardial infarction, acute coronary syndrome, maintenance of extracorporeal circuits
Heparinoid — danaparoid (contains mainly depolymerised heparan sulphate and dermatan sulphate)	Heparin-induced thrombocytopenia
Direct factor Xa inhibitor — fondaparinux and idaparinux	Prophylaxis against venous thromboembolism in high-risk orthopaedic surgery patients, heparin-induced thrombocytopenia
Direct thrombin inhibitors — argatroban, hirudins such as lepirudin (recombinant hirudin) and bivalrudin (a hirudin analogue)	Heparin-induced thrombocytopenia

Table 12.3.   Orally active anticoagulants.

Agent	Uses
Vitamin K antagonists — coumarins and indanediones	Venous thromboembolism, atrial fibrillation, prosthetic cardiac valves
Direct thrombin inhibitors — dabigatran etexilate	Venous thromboembolism, atrial fibrillation
Direct factor Xa inhibitors — rivaroxaban and apixaban	Prophylaxis against venous thromboembolism

Vitamin K antagonists

The vitamin K antagonists fall into two drug groups, the coumarins and the indanediones such as phenindione. The drug most used in the UK is warfarin, which is one of the coumarins. Vitamin K is needed for the final step in the conversion of precursors of the vitamin K-dependent coagulation factors (factors II, VII, IX and X) into their active forms. This final step, γ-carboxylation, is blocked when vitamin K deficiency or a vitamin K antagonist prevents vitamin K from being converted to its active form. The vitamin K-dependent factors are needed for both the intrinsic and the extrinsic pathways of coagulation (Fig. 12.4). However, they have a greater effect on the extrinsic than the intrinsic pathway so that a modification of the prothrombin time is used for monitoring. This test is the international normalised ratio (INR). This is a mathematical manipulation of the prothrombin time, which takes account of the difference in prothrombin times measured with different thromboplastins. Each batch of thromboplastin produced by a manufacturer is compared with an International Reference Thromboplastin and is assigned an International Sensitivity Index (ISI). The INR is then calculated as the ratio of the patient's prothrombin time to the prothrombin time of pooled normal plasma, raised to the power of the ISI.

$$\left(\frac{\text{Patient's prothrombin time}}{\text{Mean normal prothrombin time}} \right)^{\text{ISI}}$$

The time for vitamin K antagonists to have an effect depends on the plasma half-life of the various vitamin K-dependent factors. However, it

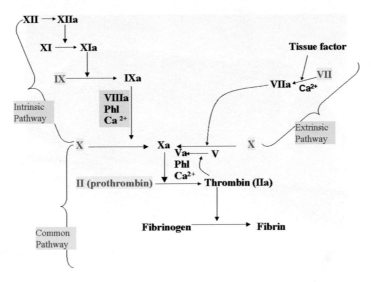

Fig. 12.4. The coagulation factors synthesis of which is affected by vitamin K-dependent factors (blue). Note that a prothrombin time will be affected by concentrations of three of these four factors.

is at least some days since it is the level of factor II, which has a long half-life, that is most important for the anticoagulant effect. When there is a need for immediately effective anticoagulation it is necessary to use heparin initially and continue it for at least 5 days; there should also be a 3-day overlap of the oral anticoagulant and heparin. In hospitalised patients, the INR is measured daily during this period until it is in the therapeutic range and it should have been in the therapeutic range for at least 2 days before stopping heparin.

Vitamin K antagonists have a narrow therapeutic window. To reduce the risk of bleeding, their effect must be carefully monitored throughout therapy and a therapeutic range appropriate to the degree of thrombotic risk must be selected. For example, an INR of 2.0–3.0 is sufficient for a patient being treated, after initial heparinisation, for a venous thrombosis or a pulmonary embolus whereas for a patient with a prosthetic cardiac valve an INR of 2.5–4.0 is usually selected.

The effect of vitamin K antagonists can be unpredictable, being influenced, for example, by diet, alcohol and the intake of drugs that interfere

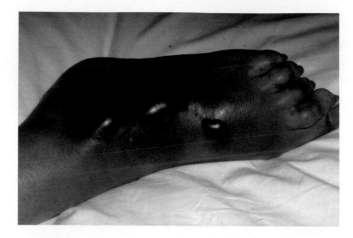

Fig. 12.5.   Haemorrhage as a result of tripping on a footpath in a patient taking warfarin for a prosthetic cardiac valve.

with the metabolism of the oral anticoagulant. Dosage requirement is lower in the elderly and in those with congestive cardiac failure or liver disease. It is therefore necessary to check the INR at least every 4–6 weeks even in a patient who is usually stable. Patients whose anticoagulant control is unstable need monitoring much more frequently.

The most frequent adverse effect of oral anticoagulant therapy is haemorrhage (Fig. 12.5). The effect on the coagulation system can be reversed by the administration of vitamin K1 either orally or intravenously. This takes several hours to be effective since coagulation factor precursors must be γ-carboxylated. More rapid reversal can be achieved by transfusion of fresh-frozen plasma or prothrombin complex.

Coumarin anticoagulants cross the placenta and are teratogenic. They should not be administered during the first trimester of pregnancy.

Direct thrombin inhibitors

Orally active direct thrombin inhibitors can be used in a similar manner to warfarin but in a fixed dose and without the need for monitoring. One of these drugs, dabigatran etexilate, has shown similar efficacy and safety to warfarin in atrial fibrillation, treatment of acute VTE and prevention of

VTE after high-risk orthopaedic surgery including total hip and knee arthroplasty.

Direct factor Xa inhibitors

Orally active direct factor Xa inhibitors, such as rivaroxaban, are of use in prophylaxis against thrombosis. Monitoring is not required.

Antiplatelet Agents

Various drugs interfere with platelet aggregation and can be used as antithrombotic agents. Their sites of action are shown in Fig. 12.6. Antiplatelet drugs with different mechanisms of action are synergistic.

Aspirin

Arachidonic acid in the platelet membrane is converted to the aggregating agent, thromboxane A2, by the consecutive actions of cyclo-oxgenase and

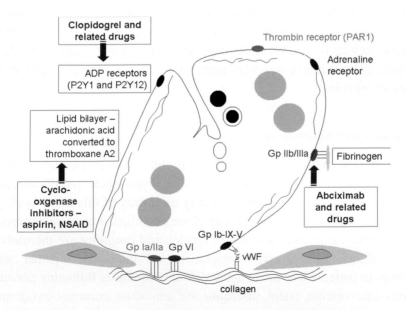

Fig. 12.6. Sites of action of different classes of antiplatelet drug (bold red). For an explanation of other parts of the diagram see Fig. 11.3.

thromboxane synthase. Aspirin acetylates and irreversibly inactivates cyclo-oxygenase. It thus causes an impairment of platelet function that persists for the life span of the platelet. In higher doses, aspirin interferes with the synthesis of endothelial cell prostacyclin and therefore when it is used as an antithrombotic agent it is used in low dose, e.g. 75 mg daily. Aspirin is indicated in patients with acute coronary syndromes and should be continued indefinitely. Its long-term use is also indicated following myocardial infarction and ischaemic stroke. Aspirin is administered to patients at risk of thrombosis because of polycythaemia vera and essential thrombocythaemia. Non-steroidal anti-inflammatory drugs (NSAID) also inhibit cyclo-oxgenase but the effect is reversible.

Aspirin therapy is associated with an increased risk of haemorrhage, particularly gastrointestinal haemorrhage. Because platelet function is impaired for the life span of the platelet, serious haemorrhage may require platelet transfusion.

Platelet phosphodiesterase inhibitors

Platelet phosphodiesterase inhibitors increase platelet cyclic adenosine monophosphate and thus inhibit platelet aggregation. They include dipyridamole, which is used for its antithrombotic effect and anagrelide, which reduces platelet production from megakaryocytes in addition to inhibiting platelet function.

ADP-receptor antagonists

Drugs of this group, or their active metabolites, antagonise platelet function by binding to the platelet adenosine diphosphate (ADP) receptor (known as P2Y12). The most frequently used drug of this group is clopidogrel. Both clopidogrel and prasugrel are prodrugs, which are converted to an active metabolite, whereas ticagrelor and cangrelor are themselves active drugs. ADP-receptor antagonists are indicated, together with aspirin, in patients who are at acute risk of thrombosis following percutaneous intervention (stent insertion) for an acute coronary syndrome. These drugs can also be used in other circumstances when aspirin therapy would be indicated but cannot be tolerated by the patient. The effects of clopidogrel and prasugrel are irreversible whereas ticagrelor and can-grelor effects are reversible.

Platelet glycoprotein IIb/IIIa fibrinogen receptor inhibitors

This group of drugs bind to the platelet fibrinogen receptor, platelet glyoprotein IIb/IIIa. They include eptifibatide, tirofiban and abciximab (a human-mouse chimaeric monoclonal antibody). They are indicated, as a supplement to aspirin and clopidogrel, in some patients with acute coronary syndromes and, briefly, following percutaneous coronary intervention. In a small percentage of patients (0.5–1%) first exposure to these drugs can lead to the sudden onset of severe thrombocytopenia.

Epoprostenol

Epoprostenol (prostacyclin) is a potent parenteral vasodilator and inhibitor of platelet aggregation. Its main use is in refractory pulmonary hypertension.

Thrombolytic Therapy

Patients who have suffered thrombosis but do not yet have irreversible tissue injury may benefit from therapeutic thrombolysis. Such patients include those with recent coronary occlusion and actual or impending myocardial infarction, and those presenting with a cerebrovascular accident and found to have cerebral thrombosis or embolism. Thrombolytic therapy should be given speedily, e.g. within 12 hours of the onset of symptoms of coronary occlusion.

In patients with primary myocardial infarction, angioplasty is the preferred procedure, supplemented by aspirin, clopidogrel and a platelet IIb/IIIa inhibitor such as abciximab. When this cannot be achieved within 90 minutes, thrombolytic therapy becomes the preferred option.

In patients with ischaemic stroke, thrombolytic therapy is indicated if there are no contraindications and if it can be given within 3 hours of the event. It is possible that treatment even up to 4.5 or 6 hours from the event may be efficacious.

In patient with thrombosed indwelling catheters, cannulae or shunts (e.g. arteriovenous shunts to permit haemodialysis), thrombolytic therapy, which can be administered at the site of thrombosis, may restore patency. Regional thrombolysis, using catheter delivery, can also be of benefit for arterial thrombosis causing critical ischaemia and venous thrombosis causing arterial compromise.

Agents that can be employed for thrombolysis include recombinant human proteins and streptokinase, which is of bacterial origin. Human products that are available include recombinant tissue plasminogen activator (alteplase) and urokinase. Complications include bleeding (especially intracranial), hypotension and allergic reactions.

Antithrombotic Management of Specific Conditions

Various anticoagulant, antiplatelet and thrombolytic agents are used alone or in combination in the management of thrombotic and thromboembolic disorders, as shown in Table 12.4. The specific choice of drugs and drug

Table 12.4.   The integration of anticoagulant, antiplatelet and thrombolytic therapy in the management of thrombotic disorders.

Conditions	Agents that are indicated
Prevention of venous thromboembolism in high-risk surgical patients	Low molecular weight heparin or possibly a direct thrombin inhibitor (dabigatran orally) or a factor Xa inhibitor (fondaparinux parenterally or rivaroxaban orally)
Treatment of deep vein thrombosis or pulmonary embolism without circulatory compromise	Low molecular weight heparin (or unfractionated heparin if there is a high risk of bleeding) + continuing warfarin (target INR 2.0–3.0) or possibly plus continuing dabigatran
Treatment of pulmonary embolism with compromised circulation	Thrombolytic therapy (alteplase, streptokinase or urokinase) followed by heparin and then continuing warfarin

(Continued)

Table 12.4. (*Continued*)

Conditions	Agents that are indicated
Acute coronary syndrome (without ST segment elevation)	Aspirin + clopidogrel + an antiplatelet glycoprotein IIb/IIIa inhibitor; aspirin and clopidogrel continued for 12 months
Myocardial infarction, percutaneous coronary intervention possible within 90 minutes	Aspirin + clopidogrel + antiplatelet glycoprotein IIb/IIIa inhibitor (abciximab) + 8 days of low molecular weight heparin; long-term aspirin + clopidogrel
Myocardial infarction, percutaneous coronary intervention not possible within 90 minutes	Thrombolytic therapy (e.g. streptokinase, alteplase, reteplase or tenecteplase) + 8 days of low molecular weight heparin; long-term aspirin + clopidogrel
Acute ischaemic stroke	Thrombolytic therapy with alteplase within 3 hours (possible useful up to 6 hours); long-term aspirin + modified release dipyridamole
Transient ischaemic attach	Long-term aspirin + modified release dipyridamole
Cardiopulmonary bypass	Unfractionated heparin
Haemodialysis	Unfractionated heparin
Prosthetic heart valve	Lifelong warfarin (target INR 2.5–4.0); dipyridamole can be used as an adjunct
Tissue valve	Warfarin for 3 months (target INR 2.0–3.0)
Atrial fibrillation	Warfarin (target INR 2.0–3.0) or possibly dabigatran

combinations changes over time as results of new randomised trials become available. This table should therefore be regarded only as a guide and should be supplemented by reference to the British National Formulary and to National Institute for Health and Clinical Excellence (NICE) guidelines.

Conclusions

Thrombotic disease is a major problem in the developed world. All antithrombotic and fibrinolytic therapy requires a balancing of potential benefits and potential harm. A great variety of drugs based on different principles are available. Which are chosen in an individual patient should be based on the best evidence available, which is likely to change with time.

Test Case 12.1

A 27-year-old woman presents with swelling and tenderness of the left calf. Doppler examination shows a left deep vein thrombosis with some extension into the thigh. The patient is not taking the oral contraceptive and there are no obvious precipitating factors for a venous thrombosis. She has not attended her GP for some time but on specific questioning she admits to intermittent joint swelling. An FBC and a coagulation screen are performed prior to planned anti-coagulant therapy show:

WBC $3.4 \times 10^9/l$

Neutrophil count $1.2 \times 10^9/l$

Hb 12.9 g/dl

Platelet count $72 \times 10^9/l$

Prothrombin time 14 sec (normal range [NR] 12–14)

Activated partial thromboplastin time 67 sec (NR 30–40)

Thrombin time 20 sec (control 21 sec)

Questions

1. What do you suspect?
2. If your suspicions are correct, what treatment is indicated?
3. Are any further investigations indicated?

Write down your answers before checking the correct answer (page 327) and re-reading any relevant part of the chapter.

13

Blood Transfusion and Haemopoietic Stem Cell Transplantation

What Do You Have to Know?

☞ The types of blood components and blood products that are used for transfusion

☞ How donors are recruited, screened and tested

☞ The ABO and Rh group systems and related antibodies

☞ The principles of tests done in a blood transfusion laboratory

☞ The indications for use of blood and blood products

☞ Adverse effects of blood transfusion and how specific transfusion reactions are recognised

☞ How blood transfusion can be made safer

Blood, Blood Products and Blood Components for Transfusion

Blood transfusion is crucial to the practice of modern medicine. It has made major surgery possible, has made obstetrics safer and has reduced the death rate following major trauma. It has made possible the effective treatment of inherited and acquired bleeding disorders and malignant diseases such as leukaemia and lymphoma.

Blood for transfusion is obtained by venesection of volunteer altruistic donors (Fig. 13.1). A volume of 450 ml is taken into a plastic bag

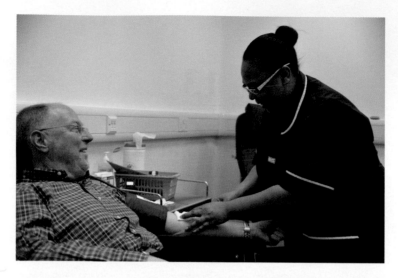

Fig. 13.1. Blood donation at a transfusion centre.

containing citrate as an anticoagulant. It is now rare for whole blood to be transfused. It is better practice to separate the blood into its components so that only what is necessary for that particular patient is transfused. The major components are red cells, plasma and platelets. Red cells either have some plasma removed (plasma-reduced red cells) or, alternatively, as much as possible of the plasma is removed and sodium chloride, adenine, glucose and mannitol (SAGM) is added to improve their survival *in vitro*. In the UK all blood is leucocyte-depleted to reduce the risk of transmission of variant Creutzfeldt-Jacob disease (vCJD).

Plasma-reduced or SAGM red cells (Fig. 13.2) can be conserved at 2–6°C for up to 35 days. This is referred to as their shelf life. Conservation at this temperature is essential to prevent bacterial proliferation. The whole blood is separated into components by centrifugation and, by means of a specialised device that compresses the bag of blood between two plates, the plasma is squeezed out at the top and the red cells at the bottom, leaving the buffy coat that contains the platelets. The platelets are resuspended in plasma, whenever possible from a male blood donor, and are depleted of white cells (leucodepleted). Platelets harvested from individual donations are pooled in a single bag; usually platelets

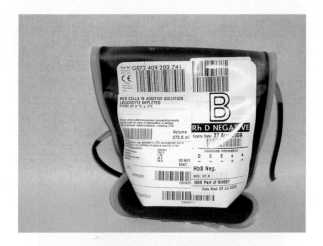

Fig. 13.2. Red cells in additive solution (SAGM red cells). The label applied by the blood transfusion service shows the blood group, the expiry date and the required storage conditions. Note that these particular red cells have also been tested for the presence of haemoglobin S, which has been found to be absent. It has also been tested for high titre ABO antibodies and the Kell antigen and has therefore been labelled NEG: HT, K. This bag of blood has not yet been cross-matched. Once this is done another label is applied showing the recipient's full name, date of birth, gender and hospital or NHS number. This second label is cross-checked with the patient's wrist band and with the request form for the blood at the bedside prior to transfusion.

from four donors are pooled (Fig. 13.3). Platelets have a better shelf life if conserved at 20–24°C and kept in motion on an agitator. Even so their shelf life is only 5 days. Plasma is frozen rapidly, this component being called fresh-frozen plasma because the plasma is frozen while it is still fresh. Taking this action means that the coagulation factors contained in the plasma remain active and fresh-frozen plasma can thus be used to treat patients with bleeding disorders. When stored at −30°C, the shelf life is 2 years.

Other blood components are also sometimes prepared from whole blood. These include granulocyte concentrates and cryoprecipitate. Granulocyte concentrates are occasionally useful in treating life-threatening infection in severely immunosuppressed patients. They are obtained as buffy coats removed from the top of the red cells after centrifugation. They contain significant numbers of red cells and have to be ABO and Rh D compatible

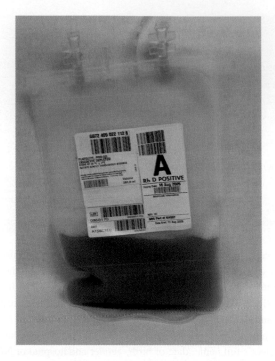

Fig. 13.3. A platelet concentrate. Note that there is some contamination with red cells. This is why platelets should be Rh D compatible, particularly in girls and women in the reproductive age range. It is also desirable for them to be ABO identical with the recipient since anti-A and anti-B in platelet concentrates can cause haemolysis.

and to be cross-matched. All buffy coats are also irradiated. Cryoprecipitate is a component made by freezing plasma and then allowing it to thaw at 4–8°C overnight. The cryoprecipitate is the residue that does not redissolve on slow thawing. It is separated from most of the plasma and stored at −30°C until needed. Cryoprecipitate contains factor VIII, von Willebrand factor and fibrinogen. It is useful for treating patients with disseminated intravascular coagulation and can be used for treating specific coagulation abnormalities, e.g. deficiency of fibrinogen or von Willebrand factor.

Blood components can also be obtained by component donation, using the process of apheresis. A volunteer component donor is attached to a cell separator machine by two intravenous lines, one which takes the blood from the donor to the machine and another which returns blood,

Table 13.1. (*Continued*)

Component or product	Major therapeutic role	Provisos and comments
Albumin	Hypoproteinaemia, burns, plasma exchange	Has been pasteurised so does not transmit viruses
Immunoglobulin	Correction of deficiency; in high doses, for treatment of autoimmune diseases (such as autoimmune thrombocytopenic purpura)	
Factor VIII concentrate	Treatment of haemophilia A and von Willebrand disease	For haemophilia A, recombinant factor VIII is preferred, when available
Factor IX concentrate	Treatment of haemophilia B	Recombinant factor IX is preferred, when available
Prothrombin complex concentrate (factors II, IX, X and possibly VII)	Correction of deficiency including haemorrhage resulting from coumarin therapy	
Antithrombin	Correction of deficiency	

*Massive blood loss can be defined as blood loss equalling or exceeding one blood volume in 24 hours, the normal adult blood volume being approximately 7% of ideal body weight; alternative definitions include loss of 50% of blood volume within 3 hours or, for an adult, blood loss at a rate exceeding 150 ml/minute.

They are absent at birth but develop following exposure to environmental antigens. They are mainly immunoglobulin (Ig) M, are reactive at 37°C and can activate complement. Some individuals also have IgG antibodies, particularly if they have received certain vaccinations. If a transfusion accident occurs and ABO-incompatible blood is given, intravascular haemolysis, which can be life-threatening, occurs. In addition, IgG antibodies can cross the placenta and can cause ABO haemolytic disease of the newborn, e.g. if an O mother has an A or B fetus.

The Rh blood group system has five possible antigens at two closely linked loci, the D locus and the CcEe locus. Of these, the most important antigen is D. Among the UK population, 85% of individuals are D-positive

Table 13.2. Requirements that must be met by a volunteer blood donor in the United Kingdom.*

Requirement	Comment
Age between 17 and 70 (or 17 to 60 for a first-time donor)	For the protection of the donor
In good health, weighing at least 50 kg, normal blood pressure, on no medications that might be harmful to the recipient	For the protection of the donor and the recipient: medications present in the plasma can have adverse effects in the recipient
Haemoglobin concentration at least 13.5 g/l in a man and at least 12.5 g/dl in a woman	For the protection of the donor
Has not been transfused since 1st January 1980 and did not receive human pituitary extract pre-1985	Risk that potential donor has acquired prions of new variant Creutzfeldt-Jacob disease
Has not visited a malaria zone during the previous 6 months (or anti-malaria antibodies are absent at 6 months)	Risk of malaria
Has not visited Central or South America for a period of 4 weeks or more (or antibodies to *T. cruzi* are negative)	Risk of Chagas' disease
No history of intravenous drug use	Risk of HIV
Has not had sex with another man at any time since 1977	Risk of HIV
Has not lived in an African country, except those bordering the Mediterranean, since 1977	Risk of HIV
Has not acted as a prostitute (man or woman)	Risk of HIV
Has not had acupuncture, ear piercing, body piercing, tattooing or semi-permanent make-up in the previous 4 months	Risk of blood-born viruses

Abbreviation: HIV — human immunodeficiency virus.

*These requirements are not exhaustive. For a donor questionnaire see www.blood.co.uk.

Table 13.3. Tests performed on donor blood in the United Kingdom to reduce the risk of transmission of infectious agents.*

Infectious agent	Tests
Treponema pallidum (syphilis)	Serology
Hepatitis B	Hepatitis B surface antigen
Hepatitis C	Serology and hepatitis C RNA
Human T-cell lymphotropic virus I	Serology
Human immunodeficiency virus	Serology for HIV1 and HIV2 and HIV RNA

Abbreviations: HIV — human immunodeficiency virus; RNA — ribonucleic acid.

*In addition, selected units are tested for antibodies to cytomegalovirus, malaria and *Trypanosoma cruzi*.

Table 13.4. The ABO blood group system.

Blood group	Genotype	Frequency in the UK population	ABO antigens present	ABO antibodies present*
O	OO	46%	None	Anti-A and anti-B
A	AA or AO	43%	A	Anti-B
B	BB or BO	8%	B	Anti-A
AB	AB	3%	A and B	None

*ABO antibodies are absent in neonates and in patients with agammaglobulinaemia.

(also referred to as Rh positive and previously as Rhesus positive). The 15% who are D-negative are designated dd but it should be noted that d is not an antigen, merely the absence of a gene encoding D at one or both allelic loci. D is necessarily dominant so a D-positive person may be DD or Dd. D-negative individuals can develop anti-D if they are exposed to D-positive cells, either by transfusion or by transplacental transfer of red cells from a fetus to a pregnant woman. Anti-D antibodies are important because they can cross the placenta and lead to haemolytic disease of the fetus and newborn in an Rh D-positive baby. They can also lead to a delayed transfusion reaction if D-positive red cells are transfused into a D-negative individual who has previously been exposed to the D antigen; the antibody level is boosted (from undetectable levels to clinically significant levels) by the transfusion leading to extravascular haemolysis.

Antibodies can also develop against C, c, E and e but these are less often a problem and generally blood for transfusion is selected without considering these antigens. However, blood for girls or women of childbearing potential is selected to be K negative to prevent development of anti-K which can cause severe haemolytic disease of the newborn.

Haemolytic disease of the newborn

IgG antibodies can cross the placenta and bind to antigens on fetal cells, leading to haemolytic disease of the fetus or the newborn (HDFN). Anti-D antibodies can cause serious HDFN which, if not correctly managed, can cause death *in utero* or soon after birth from anaemia-induced hydrops fetalis. Following birth, brain damage can occur if the plasma bilirubin is permitted to rise above a safe level; this is known as kernicterus and results from binding of bilirubin to the basal ganglia. Because of the serious consequences, management during pregnancy and after birth is in specialist centres. IgG anti-A or anti-B cause haemolytic disease mainly in the newborn (HDN). Naturally occurring IgM antibodies of the ABO system cannot cross the placenta so do not cause HDN.

Management of haemolytic disease of the fetus and newborn

Management of ABO HDN is by exposure to light from the blue end of the spectrum (phototherapy). This leads to isomerisation of bilirubin and enhances its clearance without the need for conjugation; bilirubin concentration can thus be controlled. Rarely, exchange transfusion is needed. Management of Rh D HDFN is complex and should be done at a specialist centre. Intrauterine transfusion may be required. Non-invasive monitoring of middle cerebral artery blood flow is used to predict fetal anaemia and the need for transfusion. Following birth, phototherapy and exchange transfusion may be needed.

Prevention of haemolytic disease of the fetus and newborn

Women may develop anti-D antibodies as a result of transfusion of D-positive blood components or by sensitisation during pregnancy.

Sensitisation is the result of small amounts of D-positive fetal blood crossing into the maternal circulation, particularly at delivery but also during pregnancy. Certain events during pregnancy increase the likelihood of sensitisation (Box 13.1).

Box 13.1
Sensitisation to D antigen may occur as a result of

Spontaneous miscarriage
Termination of pregnancy
Ectopic pregnancy
Chorionic villus sampling
Amniocentesis or cordocentesis
Abdominal trauma
External version of the fetus
Antepartum haemorrhage
Delivery (higher risk with caesarean section than normal delivery)

Sensitisation can largely be prevented by administration of anti-D Ig to D-negative women who are or might be carrying a D-positive fetus. In the UK, routine antenatal anti-D prophylaxis is given in the last trimester. Regimes vary but either a dose of at least 500 international units (iu) of anti-D Ig is given at 28 and 34 weeks gestation or, alternatively, a single 1500 iu dose is given at 28–30 weeks gestation.

A further dose of at least 500 iu is given as soon as possible after delivery but always within 72 hours to mothers of D-positive babies. Before the post-partum dose is given, a maternal blood sample should be taken to quantitate any detectable fetomaternal haemorrhage in case a larger than standard dose of anti-D is needed. A standard dose of anti-D must be given whenever there is a D-negative mother with a D-positive baby, even if no fetomaternal haemorrhage is detected. Anti-D is also given as soon as possible after the occurrence of high-risk events during pregnancy and again must be given within 72 hours of the event. Administered anti-D prevents the immune system from recognising D-positive red cells as foreign.

Rh D-positive blood components must never be given to girls or women of childbearing potential. If this inadvertently occurs, exchange transfusion and administration of large doses of anti-D may prevent sensitisation.

ABO HDN can occur in the first pregnancy and no method of prevention is known.

Tests Done in a Blood Transfusion Laboratory

Tests done by a hospital transfusion laboratory are: (i) blood grouping of patients who may require transfusion; (ii) screening of the plasma of potential transfusion recipients for atypical blood group antibodies; (iii) cross-matching; and (iv) testing for the detection of transfusion reactions and for the diagnosis of autoimmune haemolytic anaemia. The purpose of most transfusion laboratory procedures is the provision of compatible blood for transfusion.

Blood grouping

The blood grouping of a potential transfusion recipient requires determining the ABO and Rh D groups. The ABO group is determined by testing the cells with reagents containing saline-reacting monoclonal anti-A or anti-B antibodies; this is known as the forward group. In addition, the patient's plasma is tested against reagent red cells to detect anti-A and anti-B in the patient's plasma and thus confirm that the grouping of the red cells was correct; this is known as the reverse group Expected reactions are shown in Fig. 13.4. The Rh D group is determined with two different anti-D reagents to lessen the chance of error. Patients who are going to be regularly transfused, for example for beta thalassaemia major or sickle cell disease, may be grouped for a wider range of red cell antigens. Blood can then be selected that is less likely to lead to the development of antibodies that will interfere with future transfusion. Such extended phenotyping is usually for CcEe and K.

Antibody screening

Unless the transfusion is urgent, the transfusion recipient's plasma is tested for atypical red cell antibodies, i.e. antibodies other than the expected anti-A

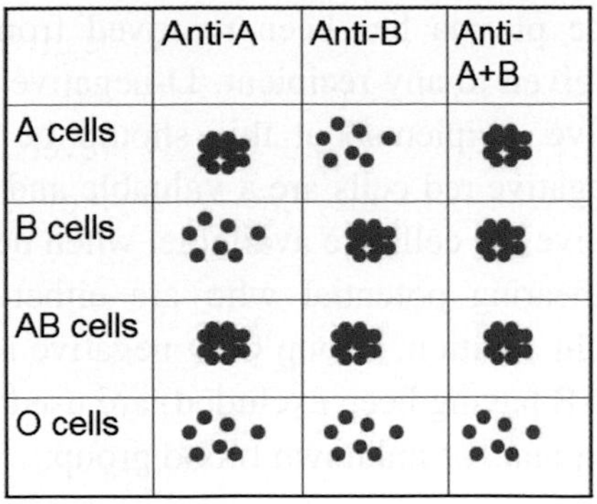

	Anti-A	Anti-B	Anti-A+B
A cells	✸	∴	✸
B cells	∴	✸	✸
AB cells	✸	✸	✸
O cells	∴	∴	∴

Fig. 13.4. A diagram showing expected reactions in ABO blood grouping. When an IgM antibody that is present in the plasma binds to an antigen on the red blood cells, a tight agglutinate is formed (e.g. A cells with anti-A). When no such antibody is present cells remain dispersed (e.g. A cells with anti-B).

or anti-B, using a panel of three well-characterised screening cells on which are represented all antigens that are likely to be important in a transfusion reaction. If an antibody is found it is characterised using a panel of reagent red cells selected for the purpose of antibody identification. It is then possible to select blood that lacks that relevant antigen as well as cross-matching donor red cells against the patient's plasma.

Cross-matching

If a patient's blood group has been determined on two separate blood specimens and if atypical antibodies have been excluded it is not necessary to cross-match blood. Blood of a suitable group can be issued electronically. This is sometimes referred to as an electronic cross-match but the preferred term is electronic issue since no actual cross-match has been performed. If an antibody screen has not been done, if an atypical antibody has been detected or if the blood group has been determined on only one specimen, cross-matching, in which the patient's plasma is tested with donor red cells, is obligatory.

Compatible blood does not have to be identical, e.g. group B red cells could be transfused into a group AB recipient. From Table 13.4 you will be able to work out which red cells are suitable for recipients of various blood groups. Since plasma has been removed from donor red cells, O red cells can be given to any recipient. D-negative cells can be transfused into D-positive recipients but this should be avoided as far as possible since D-negative red cells are a valuable and scarce resource. It is vital that D-negative red cells are available, when needed, for girls and women with childbearing potential who are either D-negative or of unknown D group. In addition, Group O D-negative red cells (with high titre anti-A and anti-B having been excluded) are used in emergencies for transfusion into recipients of unknown blood group.

Investigation of a suspected transfusion reaction or suspected autoimmune haemolytic anaemia

If an incompatible transfusion is suspected as the cause of a transfusion reaction the transfusion is stopped immediately and further laboratory tests are done. The blood group of the patient and the donor unit are re-checked and an antibody screen is performed (or is repeated if already done). In addition, a direct antiglobulin test is performed, to detect any antibody or complement on the surface of circulating red cells (which would suggest that a recipient antibody has bound to donor cells). The principles of the direct antiglobulin test, also referred to as a Coombs' test, are shown in Fig. 13.5. A direct antiglobulin test is also important in investigating suspected autoimmune haemolytic anaemia.

There are other types of transfusion reaction, which are summarised later in Tables 13.5 and 13.6.

The Indications for Blood Transfusion

The only indications for red cell transfusion are correction of anaemia and replacement of blood that has been or is being lost. There are further indications for exchange transfusion, including HDN and some complications of sickle cell anaemia. Despite the efforts of all concerned, blood transfusion is never totally free of risk. It is therefore essential that blood components are only transfused when there is a clear clinical need and there is no safer alternative. For example, a patient with anaemia might respond to iron or erythropoietin or it might be possible during surgery to

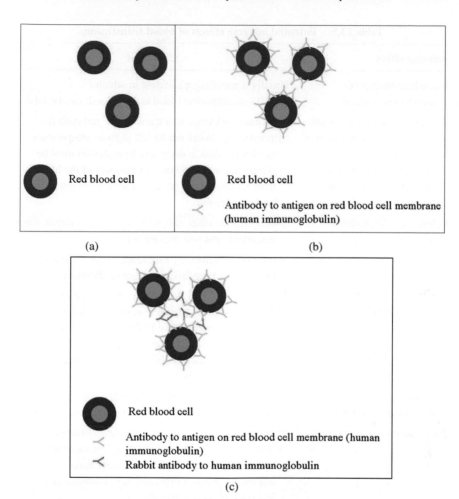

Fig. 13.5. The principle of a direct antiglobulin (Coombs') test: **(a)** red cells are separate in the plasma and there is no antibody bound to them (the normal state); **(b)** a non-agglutinating antibody is present and has bound to an antigen on the red cells (the cells are 'sensitised' but are still separate from each other); **(c)** the cells are washed to remove free antibody and a rabbit antibody to human immunoglobulin is added. The rabbit antibody binds to the human immunoglobulin that is already bound to the antigen on the red cell surface membrane, thus cross-linking the cells and causing them to agglutinate; the presence of the non-agglutinating primary antibody is now revealed by the visible agglutination of the cells. The human antibody that is detected may be either an alloantibody, if there has been a transfusion reaction, or an autoantibody, if the patient has autoimmune haemolytic anaemia. An antibody to complement can also be used to detect complement on the cell surface.

Table 13.5.   Potential adverse effects of blood transfusion.

Adverse effect	Comment
Immediate haemolytic transfusion reaction	Usually a transfusion accident in which ABO-incompatible blood is transfused; can be fatal
Transfusion-associated sepsis due to bacterial infection of red cell or platelet concentrates (particularly platelets since they are stored at room temperature)	Can cause endotoxic shock and death; red cells for transfusion should not be left at room temperature any longer than is necessary (transfusion must be completed within 5 hours of removal of the blood from refrigeration); platelets can now be tested for bacterial growth
Febrile, non-haemolytic reaction	Usually due to white cell antibodies, less common since leucodepletion was introduced
Cardiac failure	Should be prevented by avoidance of use of whole blood, slow transfusion and use of diuretics
Transfusion-related acute lung injury (TRALI)	Results from anti-HLA or antineutrophil antibodies in donor plasma; incidence is reduced by leucocyte depletion, by using only FFP from male donors and by either deriving platelet pools from male donors or re-suspended platelets from females in plasma from males; can be fatal
Delayed haemolytic transfusion reaction	Often due to Rh antibodies (e.g. anti-c), leads to jaundice and a fall of the haemoglobin concentration
Post-transfusion purpura	Platelet count falls 7–10 days after transfusion due to development of alloantibodies and an innocent bystander reaction; high-dose intravenous immunoglobulin is indicated; less common since leucodepletion was introduced
Transmission of viruses	Very rarely transmission of HIV, hepatitis B or hepatitis C occurs in the 'window period' before antibodies have developed in the donor and before there is a sufficient viral load for detection by PCR; parvovirus, Epstein–Barr virus, cytomegalovirus, human herpesvirus 8 and West Nile virus can be transmitted
Transmission of parasites	Malaria, babesiosis, trypanosomiasis, toxoplasmosis and leishmaniasis have all been transmitted

(Continued)

Table 13.5.   (*Continued*)

Adverse effect	Comment
Transmission of bacterial infections	Brucellosis, syphilis, Lyme disease (*Borrelia burgdorferi*), salmonellosis and rickettsial infections (Q fever and Rocky Mountain spotted fever) have been transmitted; *Yersinia enterocolitica* can be transmitted in white cells
Graft-versus-host disease	Can occur if viable lymphocytes are transfused into immuno-incompetent hosts; should be prevented by using only irradiated blood for vulnerable recipients; fatal
Iron overload	Occurs with chronic transfusion programmes for thalassaemia major and requires chelation therapy

Abbreviations: FFP — fresh-frozen plasma; HLA — human leucocyte antigens; PCR — polymerase chain reaction.

Table 13.6.   Clinical features suggesting a specific type of transfusion reaction.

Type of reaction	Clinical features
Immediate haemolytic transfusion reaction	Restlessness, anxiety, fever, chills, loin pain, chest tightness, nausea, vomiting, shock, haemorrhage (due to DIC), haemoglobinaemia and haemoglobinuria, subsequently renal failure
Transfusion-associated sepsis	Fever, shock, sometimes DIC or renal failure
Febrile, non-haemolytic reaction	Fever, chills, rigors; tends to recur
Allergic reaction	Itch, urticaria, peri-orbital oedema, wheeze, rash (rarely reactions are anaphylactic, e.g. in IgA-deficient patients, and these can be fatal)
Transfusion-related acute lung injury (TRALI)	Acute dyspnoea within 6 hours of transfusion, fever, tachycardia, tachypnoea, hypoxia, bilateral infiltrates on chest radiology
Delayed haemolytic transfusion reaction	Jaundice, anaemia and fever occurring from 1 to 7 days after transfusion

Abbreviations: DIC — disseminated intravascular coagulation; Ig — immunoglobulin.

salvage red cells from any clean operative site and, following washing and centrifugation, re-infuse them into the patient. Use of predeposited autologous blood can also avoid some allogeneic transfusions but it is used only in special circumstances, e.g. in a patient with a rare blood group. Similarly, in considering transfusion of platelets, guidelines should be followed to avoid unnecessary transfusion (Box 13.2).

Box 13.2
Triggers for giving a platelet transfusion in patients with normal platelet function who are not bleeding

Prophylaxis in a patient, e.g. with acute leukaemia, who is not bleeding: platelet count $\leq 10 \times 10^9/l$

Patient with serious trauma or who requires surgery: platelet count $\leq 50 \times 10^9/l$

Patient who needs neurosurgery: platelet count $\leq 100 \times 10^9/l$

The Adverse Effects of Transfusion

Adverse effects occur in a small but nevertheless significant proportion of patients who are transfused. Some of these are shown in Table 13.5 and the clinical features that permit them to be suspected are summarised in Table 13.6. Patients can be reassured that transmission of infectious agents by UK blood is very rare (Box 13.3). On average there is transmission of about two viral infections per year.

Box 13.3
Estimated risk of acquiring specified infection from one unit of UK blood

Hepatitis B	1 in 850,000
Hepatitis C	1 in 50,000 million
HIV	1 in 5 million

How Blood Transfusion Can Be Made Safer

Safe blood transfusion requires conscientious behaviour on the part of all concerned. The first step to be taken is to explain the purpose and also the risks and benefits of transfusion to the patient. The patient must agree to transfusion. A blood sample from the patient is then obtained, with the identity of the patient first being carefully checked. This is done by asking the patient to state his or her full name and date of birth and, in the case of a hospital inpatient, by checking these details on the patient's wrist band; this may be a visual check or electronic scanning. The specimen must be fully labelled. If it is not, it will be rejected by the transfusion laboratory leading to a delay in transfusion. Labelling must be done immediately, at the patient's bedside but bottles must not be labelled in advance. Bottles must not be labelled with an addressograph label unless this has been printed at the patient's bedside from the bar-coded wrist band. Correct procedures must then be followed in the laboratory. Finally, the utmost care must be taken in transfusing the right blood to the right patient. This should involve the same checks of identity that were done when the blood sample was obtained, these being compared with the patient details on the bag of blood (Fig. 13.6). Electronic scanning of the details on the wrist band and bag of blood is an alternative.

Some of the other ways of avoiding or managing adverse events are shown in Table 13.5. The risks of transfusion in babies can be reduced by ensuring that if repeated red cell transfusions are necessary they come from the same donor. This can be achieved by separating the donor unit into a number of paediatric packs containing a suitably small volume of red cells and reserving those from a single donor for an individual baby.

Plasma can have most viruses inactivated by treatment of individual donations with methylene blue. This is done for any plasma transfused into children of adolescents in the UK. The risk of transmission of viruses can also be reduced by pooling plasma into very large pools which are then solvent-detergent treated to inactivate most viruses. To reduce the possible risk of transmission of vCJD, plasma of UK origin is no longer used for fractionation nor is it used as fresh-frozen plasma for children.

Platelets can be made safer by testing for bacterial contamination but this is not currently done in the UK.

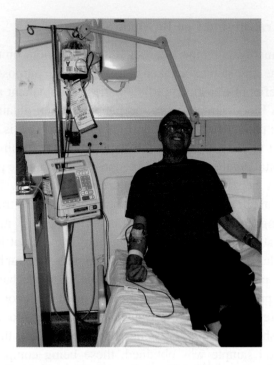

Fig. 13.6. A patient having a blood transfusion. Note that he is wearing an identifying wrist band.

Bone Marrow and Other Haemopoietic Stem Cell Transplantation

A number of haematological and non-haematological conditions can be treated by transplantation of allogeneic haemopoietic stem cells, obtained either by harvesting bone marrow or by collection of peripheral blood stem cells. Harvesting of bone marrow is done under general anaesthetic with a large needle and syringe, aspirating from multiple sites that contain red marrow, usually from multiple sites on both iliac bones. Harvesting of peripheral blood stem cells is done on a cell separator, and is made possible by the prior injection of granulocyte colony-stimulating factor (G-CSF) to mobilise stem cells from the marrow. Donor stem cells are administered intravenously and find their way to the bone marrow of the recipient. Following engraftment, they proliferate and differentiate, and repopulate the marrow with haemopoietic

Table 13.7. Some indications for haemopoietic stem cell transplantation.

Indication	Principle
Aplastic anaemia	Provision of haemopoietic stem cells
Severe combined immunodeficiency	Provision of lymphoid stem cells
β thalassaemia major	Replacement of genetically abnormal stem cells
Sickle cell anaemia	Replacement of genetically abnormal stem cells
Acute myeloid and acute lymphoblastic leukaemia	Replacement of stem cells after intensive chemotherapy has destroyed both leukaemic cells and residual normal stem cells; elimination of any residual leukaemic cells by graft-versus-leukaemia effect
Chronic myelogenous leukaemia if refractory to tyrosine kinase inhibitors	

cells. However, for 2–3 weeks following transplantation the patient is profoundly cytopenic and in need of red cell and platelet transfusion, antibiotics and nutritional support.

The purpose of transplantation may be either to provide normal haemopoietic or lymphoid stem cells when they are lacking, to replace abnormal haemopoietic cells or to rescue a patient from bone marrow failure after intensive chemotherapy for leukaemia, lymphoma or a related condition. In the treatment of haematological malignancies by allogeneic transplantation there can also be a benefit from an immune attack on leukaemic cells by transplanted immune cells, a graft-versus-leukaemia or graft-versus-tumour effect. Following transplantation, patients must be given only irradiated blood and blood products to prevent the occurrence of transfusion-associated graft-versus-host disease. Some of the current indications for transplantation are shown in Table 13.7.

Autologous stem cell transplantation

Autologous stem cell transplantation is a method of intensifying chemotherapy in refractory malignant disease. The patient is given chemotherapy and G-CSF to mobilise stem cells, which are harvested and stored. Intensive chemotherapy is then administered, following which the stored stem cells are re-infused. The full blood count recovers within approximately 2 weeks of the infusion, this being significantly faster than it would have been without the administration of stem cells. Autologous stem cell transplantation has been applied mainly to multiple myeloma and refractory lymphoma.

Donor selection and matching

Donor stem cells may come from a sibling of other close relative, an unrelated donor or a bank of cryopreserved cord blood stem cells. Single unit cord blood stem cells are suitable only for small children since they contain only a limited number of stem cells. The use of more than one unit of cord blood stem cells may make this procedure more widely applicable. Donor histocompatibility antigens are matched as closely as possible to those of the host. This is required to prevent rejection of the transplanted cells by the host's residual immune cells and also to prevent attack on the host's tissues by donor lymphocytes, an attack that gives rise to graft-versus-host disease. Acceptance of the transplanted cells by the host is facilitated by 'conditioning' to reduce host immune responses. Conditioning can be achieved by total body irradiation or chemotherapy. Less stringent matching is needed for cord blood cell transplantation as lymphocytes are immunologically naïve.

The balance between donor and host — graft-versus-host disease

Unless the transplant is from an identical twin, there will always be some histoincompatibility. Donor lymphocytes are transplanted together with donor haemopoietic stem cells and serve to reconstitute the immune system. However, donor lymphocytes can recognise host histocompatibility antigens leading to graft-versus-host disease (GVHD), which manifests clinically particularly in the skin, gastrointestinal tract and liver. Immunosuppressive treatment (ciclosporin and methotrexate) is given post-transplant to try to reduce the incidence of GVHD. If it nevertheless occurs, further immunosuppression with corticosteroids is used. Cord blood stem transplants produce less GVHD than transplants of adult stem cells.

When transplantation is done for a benign condition, such as thalassaemia major, it is not necessary to eliminate all host haemopoietic cells so conditioning can be milder. When transplantation is for a malignant condition, intensive chemotherapy is usually used. However, it is also possible to use 'reduced intensity conditioning' and rely on the graft-versus-leukaemia effect to eliminate residual leukaemic cells. If all leukaemic cells have not been eliminated (as shown, for example, by molecular studies) or overt relapse occurs, the graft-versus-leukaemia effect can be enhanced by infusion of donor lymphocytes. (Actually, donor leucocytes are infused but it is the lymphocytes that are important.)

Morbidity and mortality of transplantation

Allogeneic transplantation is associated with significant mortality, from 10 to 40% depending on the age and general health of the recipient and the closeness of tissue matching. Death may be from bacterial, fungal or viral infection of from GVHD or relapse. There is also significant morbidity.

Reduced intensity conditioning transplantation is associated with a lower morbidity and mortality and thus has made transplantation available over a wider age range and therefore also for diseases that are particularly diseases of old age, such as myelodysplastic syndromes and chronic lymphocytic leukaemia.

Conclusions

Blood transfusion is a major therapeutic modality, supporting modern medical practice. Haemopoietic stem cell transplantation has also been an important therapeutic advance, albeit being applicable to a much smaller number of patients. Both procedures have potential hazards. Prescribing and administering blood components and products must be done with a constant awareness of the risks as well as the benefits; careful attention to detail is of critical importance. Haemopoietic stem cell transplantation is inevitably a hazardous procedure, requiring meticulous medical and nursing care.

Test Case 13.1

A 64-year-old woman with myelodysplastic syndrome has not responded to erythropoietin therapy and is now receiving a transfusion of two units of red cells each 3 weeks. This procedure is being performed in the Day Case Ward. On the day in question she has received one unit of red cells uneventfully, with a furosemide injection to prevent volume overload. Fifteen minutes after transfusion of the second bag has started she complains of suddenly feeling unwell and has chest tightness and loin pain. Her blood pressure is found to have dropped and she has tachycardia.

Question

What do you think is happening and what should be done?
Write down your answers before checking the correct answer (page 328) and re-reading any relevant part of the chapter.

14

Things You Have to Know Before
You Graduate

What Do You Have to Know?

☞ How to take a clinical history

☞ How to perform a physical examination

☞ How to request laboratory tests

☞ How to interpret laboratory tests and initiate further investigation
of abnormal results

☞ How to prescribe blood components

☞ How to prescribe and monitor heparin and oral anticoagulants

☞ When to suspect a haematological disorder and how to recognise
a haematological emergency

☞ How to acquire information you do not have

☞ How to relate to a patient

There are some parts of haematology that you need to know by the time
you graduate and commence medical practice. There are others that you
do not need to know in any detail. For example, you will need to know
how to prescribe blood components and how to manage anticoagulant
therapy, since you are likely to be responsible for these, but you do not
need to know how to treat acute myeloid leukaemia. You need to know
how to acquire and assess new information when the circumstances

require and when to ask for help. Here are some of the things you need to know.

How to Take a Clinical History

As in all branches of medicine, taking a clinical history can be of crucial importance. Features in the history that may be of particular relevance to haematological conditions are shown in Table 14.1. In assessing haemostasis, a careful clinical history is a better diagnostic tool, e.g. preoperatively, than a 'coagulation screen'.

The history should include a dietary history, which may be of relevance to deficiency of iron, vitamin B_{12} or folic acid. A history of adverse reaction to fava beans should be specifically sought if glucose-6-phosphate dehydrogenase (G6PD) deficiency is possible.

A drug history should be routinely taken, and should include a history of 'alternative' medications (which may include toxic or pharmacologically

Table 14.1. Features in the clinical history of particular relevance in patients with haematological disorders.

Feature in clinical history	What may be indicated
Fatigue, dyspnoea, ankle swelling	Anaemia
Recurrent infection	Neutropenia, defective neutrophil function, inherited or acquired immune deficiency (possible acute leukaemia, myelodysplastic syndrome, multiple myeloma)
Bruising, epistaxis, bleeding gums, menorrhagia, bleeding following surgery or trauma, any other abnormal bleeding	Thrombocytopenia, inherited or acquired coagulation defect or defect of platelet function
Jaundice	Haemolysis or ineffective haemopoiesis
Dark urine	Haemolysis
Fever, night sweats, weight loss, alcohol-induced pain or cough	Lymphoma
Pruritis	Lymphoma or polycythaemia vera
Bone pain	In a child, possible acute lymphoblastic leukaemia; in an adult, possible multiple myeloma

active substances). Of particular relevance are intake of aspirin or other drugs that interfere with platelet function, recent intake of drugs that may cause haemolysis and intake of drugs that cause macrocytosis, such as zidovudine or methotrexate. Alcohol intake should always be documented, and is of particular relevance to the assessment of macrocytosis and cytopenia. Cigarette smoking should likewise be documented since this may be the cause not only of a high haemoglobin concentration but also of an increased neutrophil or lymphocyte count.

In many clinical circumstances it is important to assess the likelihood of exposure to the human immunodeficiency virus (HIV), hepatitis B and hepatitis C, all of which can cause haematological abnormalities and also be relevant to the treatment that is given for an unrelated condition.

A travel history should be taken. It is particularly relevant to the assessment of eosinophilia.

A family history should include a history of anaemia (including specifically sickle cell disease, thalassaemia, G6PD deficiency), jaundice and any bleeding disorder. It should include not only a history of the health of parents and siblings but also, because of the possibility of autosomal or X-linked inheritance in various haematological disorders, a history of the health of cousins and male relatives on the mother's side of the family. The possibility of consanguinity should be explored when this might be relevant.

The ethnic origin should be specifically documented since it may not be obvious and yet may be relevant. For example, Mediterranean ancestry might suggest thalassaemia or G6PD deficiency.

How to Perform a Physical Examination

The physical examination should be thorough so that all organ systems are evaluated. Features of particular relevance to haematological disorders include pallor, purpura, hepatomegaly, splenomegaly, lymphadenopathy and jaundice. Glossitis, angular cheilosis and koilonychia should also be noted. Joint or muscle swelling may be indicative of a bleeding disorder and swelling around the small bones of the hands and feet in children may indicate sickle cell disease. A rectal examination is relevant when iron deficiency is found in a middle-aged or elderly person. (Remember that a negative test for faecal occult blood does not exclude persistent but intermittent blood loss as a cause of iron deficiency.)

How to Request Laboratory Tests

You should know how to complete requests for laboratory tests, whether this is done on paper or electronically. Providing accurate clinical details can be very important in helping laboratory staff to assess test results and give you an informed opinion. For example, if the patient has been recently transfused, assays of serum B_{12} and red cell folate will be invalid as will testing relevant to thalassaemia or haemoglobinopathies; if the patient has been transfused at another hospital it is highly unlikely that the laboratory staff will discover this unless you tell them. Don't forget to tell the laboratory that a patient is on warfarin or heparin, or resources may be wasted in investigating a 'coagulation defect'.

Meticulous completion of a request form is particularly important in blood transfusion; not only must identifying details be correct in every detail but previous pregnancies or blood transfusion must be documented. It is important to know if the patient is currently pregnant (for example, some transfusion laboratories provide cytomegalovirus-negative blood to pregnant women) so don't forget to give this information if the patient is attending somewhere other than the antenatal clinic. If the patient is attending the antenatal clinic don't forget to give the period of gestation as this is relevant to when tests for atypical blood group antibodies are done.

How to Interpret Laboratory Tests

You should understand the concept of a reference range and a normal range and be able to interpret tests in relation to a range provided. You should be aware of the influence of age, gender, ethnic origin and pregnancy on common haematology tests. You should be able to assess whether an abnormal test result is likely to indicate a serious disorder and whether investigation is indicated. If further investigation is indicated, you should be able to plan a cost-effective and clinically relevant sequence of testing.

How to Prescribe Blood Components

You should understand when it is appropriate to prescribe blood components and be able to do so. This includes obtaining consent for transfusion.

How to Prescribe and Monitor Anticoagulant Therapy

You should know how to prescribe unfractionated and low molecular weight heparin and oral anticoagulants and how to monitor and adjust the dose of unfractionated heparin and oral anticoagulants. This will usually be done according to guidelines available in individual hospitals but you should understand the principles.

Don't forget to plan ahead if a patient on anticoagulant therapy is going to require surgery.

When to Suspect a Haematological Disorder and How to Recognise a Haematological Emergency

There are a small number of haematological emergencies that must be recognised since delayed diagnosis can be very detrimental to the patient. These include acute promyelocytic leukaemia and other causes of disseminated intravascular coagulation and very high-grade lymphomas (such as Burkitt lymphoma). If there is reason to suspect these conditions ask for advice immediately; don't wait till the next morning. Severe thrombocytopenia also needs to be dealt with urgently but not necessarily by platelet transfusion. If the cause might be autoimmune thrombocytopenic purpura or thrombotic thrombocytopenic purpura, seek advice immediately.

Neutropenic sepsis is also a medical emergency. This may occur following cytotoxic chemotherapy in haematology or oncology patients. The units responsible will have therapeutic guidelines as to choice of antibiotics but if you are responsible for the immediate care of the patients, e.g. out-of-hours, make sure that there is no delay in taking specimens for culture and instituting antibiotic therapy. Starting treatment in such patients should take precedence over less urgent matters as death can occur rapidly when the body's defences are inadequate.

Generally, you will be aware when a haematological disorder is likely but there are some conditions that are overlooked because they are uncommon. Don't forget that swelling of a joint may be the result of undiagnosed haemophilia rather than septic arthritis, osteomyelitis or trauma. Think of haemophilia also if you are considering a diagnosis of non-accidental injury in a child who presents with bruising or bleeding. Don't forget to request a blood film in any child presenting with renal impairment, particularly if there is also jaundice, since this may be haemolytic uraemic syndrome and in an adult presenting with acute renal failure don't forget that multiple myeloma is responsible for a significant proportion of cases. In an adult any combination of anaemia, backache and renal impairment may be due to myeloma. In any patient presenting with jaundice, remember that this may represent haemolysis rather than hepatic or post-hepatic jaundice.

How to Acquire Information You Do Not Have

Your medical course should have equipped you to acquire new information when there is something you do not know. This will include obtaining information from more experienced colleagues, not only medical colleagues but also nursing staff, pharmacists and laboratory scientists. A modicum of humility does not go amiss in dealing with non-medical colleagues; they will often know a great deal that you do not know.

You should also know how to acquire specific information — from textbooks, journals and websites. You should be aware of reliable sources on information, such as the British National Formulary and the guidelines provided by The National Institute for Health and Clinical Excellence (NICE) and various professional groups (e.g. The British Committee for Standards in Haematology). Although you will not initially be making major clinical decisions unaided, you should be able to assess the validity and clinical relevance of published trials and know how to evaluate and make use of systematic reviews including meta-analyses. In assessing original articles and systematic reviews it is important not only to assess the quality of the publication but also to ask yourself two questions. Are these results applicable to my patients? Are any benefits demonstrated worth the potential harm and the cost?

How to Relate to a Patient

All patients should be treated with respect. Patients, particularly middle-aged and elderly patients, should not be addressed by their first names. Be careful not to discuss clinical matters in lifts, hospital canteens or any other place where you may be overheard. Be honest with your patients but don't force on them more information than they wish to receive. Try to present information in an optimistic manner but without concealing the truth — a difficult balance to strike. Don't be afraid to say that you don't know.

Conclusions

The skills you need to deal with haematological disorders are exactly the same skills that you need for any other branch of medicine. However, it is important to know how to deal with common haematological disorders, how to recognise an emergency and when to suspect an uncommon but important condition.

15

Further Reading

This list is provided for reference purposes and for in-depth reading of selected topics.

General

Hoffbrand, A.V., Catovsky D., Tuddenham E.G.D., *et al.* (2010). (eds), *Postgraduate Haematology, 6th Edn*, Blackwell Publishing, Oxford.

Bain, B.J. (2006). *Haemoglobinopathy Diagnosis, 2nd Edn*, Blackwell Publishing, Oxford. — includes thalassaemias (Chapter 3 of this book) and sickle cell anaemia (Chapter 5 of this book).

Bain, B.J. (2010). *Leukaemia Diagnosis, 4th Edn*, Blackwell Publishing, Oxford. — includes the myelodysplastic syndromes (Chapter 6 of this book) and leukaemias and lymphomas (Chapter 8 of this book).

www.bloodmed.com a postgraduate haematology educational website with a special section for undergraduates, British Society for Haematology and Wiley–Blackwell.

www.pbs.org/wnet/redgold information on blood and blood transfusion from USA Public Broadcast System (includes video clips and quiz).

http://teachingcases.hematology.org/ American Society of Hematology teaching cases for students.

1. Physiology of the Blood and Bone Marrow

Guo, Y., Lübbert, M. and Engelhardt, M. (2003). CD34-Stem Cells: Current Concepts and Controversies, *Stem Cells*, **21**, pp. 15–20.

Fleming, R.E. and Bacon, B.R. (2005). Orchestration of Iron Homeostasis, *N Engl. J Med*, **352**, pp. 1741–1742.

Kemna, E.H.J.M., Tjalsma, H., Willems H.L. *et al.* (2008). Hepcidin: From Discovery to Differential Diagnosis, *Haematologica*, **93**, pp. 90–97. http://www.haematologica.it/cgi/content/full/93/1/90

Ganz, T., Olbina, G., Girelli D. *et al.* (2008). Immunoassay for Human Serum Hepcidin, *Blood*, **112**, pp. 4292–4297.

2. The Blood Count and Film

Bain, B.J. (2004). *A Beginner's Guide to Blood Cells, 2nd Edn*, Blackwell Publishing, Oxford.

3. Microcytic Anaemias and the Thalassaemias

Fleming, R.E. and Bacon, B.R. (2005). Orchestration of Iron Homeostasis, *N Engl. J Med*, **352**, pp. 1741–1742.

Umbreit, J. (2005). Iron Deficiency: a Concise Review. *Am J Hematol*, **78**, pp. 225–231.

http://www.bsg.org.uk/images/stories/docs/clinical/guidelines/sbn/iron_def.pdf British Society of Gastroenterology Guidelines for the management of iron deficiency anaemia.

http://www.ironcurriculum.esh.org/ European School of Haematology, Curriculum in Iron Metabolism and Related Disorders.

http://www.cks.nhs.uk/anaemia_iron_deficiency/ NHS Clinical Knowledge summaries, iron deficiency.

Weiss, G. and Goodnough, L.T. (2005). Medical Progress: Anemia of Chronic Disease. *N Engl. J Med*, **352**, pp. 1011–1023.

4. Macrocytic Anaemias

Wickramasinghe, S.N. (2006). Diagnosis of Megaloblastic Anaemias. *Blood Rev*, **20**, pp. 299–318.

Carmel, R. (2008). How I treat Cobalamin (vitamin B$_{12}$) Deficiency. *Blood*, **112**, pp. 2214–2221.

Devalia, V. (2006). Diagnosing Vitamin B-12 Deficiency on the Basis of Serum B-12 Assay. *BMJ*, **333**, pp. 385–486.

http://www.nice.org.uk/nicemedia/pdf/CG86FullGuideline.pdf National Institute of Health and Clinical Excellence, Recognition and assessment of coeliac disease, 2009.

5. Haemoglobinopathies and Haemolytic Anaemias

Serjeant, G.R. and Sergeant, B.E. (2001). *Sickle Cell Disease, Third Edn,* Oxford University Press, Oxford.

Machado, R.F. and Gladwin, M.T. (2005). Chronic Sickle Cell Lung Disease: New Insights into the Diagnosis, Pathogenesis and Treatment of Pulmonary Hypertension, *Br J Haematol*, **129**, pp. 449–464.

Steinberg, M.H. (2005). Predicting Clinical Severity in Sickle Cell Anaemia, *Br J Haematol*, **129**, pp. 465–481.

Almeida, A. and Roberts, I. (2005). Bone Involvement in Sickle Cell Disease, *Br J Haematol*, **129**, pp. 482–490.

Solomon, L.R. (2008). Treatment and Prevention of Pain Due to Vaso-occlusive Crises in Adults with Sickle Cell Disease: an Educational Void, *Blood*, **111**, pp. 997–1003.

Bolton-Maggs, P.H., Stephens, R.F., Dodd, N.J., *et al.* (2004). General Haematology Task Force of the British Committee for Standards in Haematology. Guidelines for the Diagnosis and Management of Hereditary Spherocytosis, *Br J Haematol*, **126**, pp. 455–474.

Luzzatto, L. (2006). Glucose-6-phosphate Dehydrogenase Deficiency: From Genotype to Phenotype, *Haematologica*, **91**, pp. 1303–1306.

http://www.haematologica.it/cgi/reprint/91/10/1303

Beutler, E. (2008). Glucose-6-phosphate Dehydrogenase Deficiency: a Historical Perspective. *Blood*, **111**, pp. 16–24.

www.chime.ucl.ac.uk/APoGI/ Accessible Publishing of Genetic Information, University College and Whittington Hospital NHS Trust, information on haemoglobinopathies.

6. Miscellaneous Anaemias, Pancytopenia and the Myelodysplastic Syndromes

http://www.nice.org.uk/CG39 National Collaborating Centre for Chronic Conditions. (2006). Anaemia Management in Chronic Kidney Disease: National Clinical Guideline for Management in Adults and Children, Royal College of Physicians, London.

Marsden, P.A. (2009). Treatment of Anemia in Chronic Kidney Disease — Strategies Based on Evidence, *N Engl. J Med*, **361**, pp. 2089–2090.

Young, N.S., Calado, R.T. and Scheinberg, P. (2006). Current Concepts in the Pathophysiology and Treatment of Aplastic Anemia, *Blood*, **108**, pp. 2509–2519.

Nimer, S.D. (2008). Myelodysplastic Syndromes. *Blood*, **111**, pp. 4841–4851.

Tefferi, A. and Vardiman, J.W. (2009). Myelodysplastic Syndromes, *N Engl. J Med*, **361**, pp. 1872–1885.

Stone, R.M. (2009). How I Treat Patients with Myelodysplastic Syndromes, *Blood*, **113**, pp. 6296–6303.

7. Leucocytosis, Leucopenia and Reactive Changes in White Cells

Peterson, L. and Hrisinko, M.A. (1993). Benign Lymphocytosis and Reactive Neutrophilia. Laboratory Features Provide Diagnostic Clues, *Clin Lab. Med*, 13, pp. 863–877.

Chetham, M.M. and Roberts K.B. (1991). Infectious Mononucleosis in Adolescents. *Paediatr Ann*, 20, pp. 206–213.

Fletcher, S. and Bain, B. (2007). Diagnosis and Treatment of Hypereosinophilic Syndromes, *Curr Opin. Hematol*, 14, pp. 37–42.

8. Leukaemias and Lymphomas

Pui, C.H. and Evans, W.E. (2006). Treatment of Acute Lymphoblastic Leukemia, *N Engl. J Med*, **354**, pp. 166–178.

Pulte, D., Gondos, A. and Brenner, H. (2009). Improvement in Survival in Younger Patients with Acute Lymphoblastic Leukemia from the 1980s to the Early 21st century, *Blood*, **113**, pp. 1408–1411.

Wang, Z-Y. and Chen, Z. (2008). Acute Promyelocytic Leukemia: from Highly Fatal to Highly Curable, *Blood*, **111**, pp. 2505–2515.

Savage, D.G., Szydlo, R.M. and Goldman J.M. (1997). Clinical features at diagnosis in 430 patients with chronic myeloid leukaemia seen at a referral centre over a 16-year period, *Br J Haematol*, **96**, pp. 111–116.

Hiddemann, W., Buske, C., Dreyling, M., *et al.* (2006). Current Management of Follicular Lymphomas, *Br J Haematol*, **136**, pp. 191–202.

9. Polycythaemia, Thrombocytosis and the Myeloproliferative Neoplasms

McMullin, M.F., Bareford, D., Campbell, P., *et al.* On behalf of the General Haematology Task Force of the British Committee for Standards in Haematology. (2005). Guidelines for the Diagnosis, Investigation and Management of Polycythaemia/Erythrocytosis, *Br J Haematol*, **130**, pp. 166–173.

Harrison, C.N. (2005). Essential Thrombocythaemia: Challenges and Evidence-based Management, *Br J Haematol*, **130**, pp. 153–165.

Tefferi, A, (2000). Myelofibrosis with Myeloid Metaplasia. *N Engl. J Med*, **342**, pp. 1255–1265.

Cervantes, F. (2005). Modern Management of Myelofibrosis. *Br J Haematol*, **128**, pp. 583–592.

10. Multiple Myeloma

Kyle, W. and Rajkumar, S.V. (2008). Multiple Myeloma. *Blood*, **111**, pp. 2962–2972.

UK Myeloma Forum, British Committee for Standards in Haematology. (2001). Guideline: Diagnosis and Management of Multiple Myeloma, *Br J Haematol*, **115**, pp. 522–540.

Kyle, R.A. and Rajkumar, S.V. (2006). Monoclonal Gammopathy of Undetermined Significance, *Brit J Haematol*, **134**, pp. 573–589.

11. Platelets, Coagulation and Haemostasis

Dahlbäck, B. (2005). Blood Coagulation and its Regulation by Anticoagulant Pathways: Genetic Pathogenesis of Bleeding and Thrombotic Diseases, *J Intern. Med*, **257**, pp. 209–223.

Chee, Y.L., Crawford, J.C., Watson H.G. *et al.* (2008). Guidelines on the Assessment of Bleeding Risk Prior to Surgery or Invasive Procedures. British Committee for Standards in Haematology. *Br J Haematol*, **140**, pp. 496–504.

Cines, D.B. and Blanchette, V.S. (2002). Medical Progress: Immune Thrombocytopenic Purpura, *N Engl. J Med*, 346, pp. 998–1008.

British Committee for Standards in Haematology General Haematology Task Force. (2003). Guidelines for the Investigation and Management of Idiopathic Thrombocytopenic Purpura in Adults, Children and in Pregnancy, *Br J Haematol*, 120, pp. 574–596.

Wakentin, T.E. (2007). Drug-induced Immune-mediated Thrombocytopenia — from Purpura to Thrombosis, *N Engl. J Med*, 356, pp. 892–893.

http://www.hemostasiscme.org/ Educational website.

http://www.pathologyoutlines.com/coagulation.html Pathology educational website.

12. Thrombosis and Its Management — Anticoagulant, Antiplatelet and Thrombolytic Therapy

Baglin, T.P., Keeling, D.M. and Watson, H.G. for the British Committee for Standards in Haematology (2006). Guidelines on Oral Anticoagulation (Warfarin): 3rd edn — 2005 update, *Br J Haematol*, **132**, pp. 277–285.

Baglin, T., Barrowcliffe, T.W., Cohen, A. *et al.* (2006). Guideline on the Use and Monitoring of Heparin, *Br J Haematol*, **133**, pp. 19–34.

Francis, C.W. (2007). Prophylaxis for Thromboembolism in Hospitalized Medical patients, *N Engl. J Med*, **356**, pp. 1438–1444.

Greer, I.A. (1999). Thrombosis in Pregnancy: Maternal and Fetal Issues. *Lancet*, **353**, pp. 1258–1264.

Reitsma, P.H. and Rosendaal, F.R. (2007). Past and Future of Genetic Research in Thrombosis, *J Thromb. Haemostas*, **5**, pp. 264–269.

Lijfering, W.M., Brouwer, J.L., Veeger, N.J., *et al.* (2009). Selective Testing for Thrombophilia in Patients with Venous Thrombosis: Results from a

Retrospective Family Cohort Study of Absolute Thrombotic Risk for Currently Known Thrombophilic Defects in 2479 Relatives, *Blood*, **113**, pp. 5314–5322.

Hillis, L.D. and Lange, R.A. (2009). Optimal Management of Acute Coronary Syndromes, *N Engl. J Med*, **360**, pp. 2237–2240.

Wakentin, T.E. (2007). Drug-induced Immune-mediated Thrombocytopenia — from Purpura to Thrombosis, *N Engl. J Med*, **356**, pp. 892–893.

Giannakopoulos, B., Passam, F., Ioannou, Y., *et al.* (2009). How we Diagnose the Antiphospholipid Syndrome, *Blood*, **113**, pp. 985–994.

http://www.nice.org.uk/nicemedia/pdf/CG68FullGuideline.pdf National Clinical Guideline for Diagnosis and Initial Management of Acute Stroke and Transient Ischaemic Attack (TIA). (2008). National Institute of Health and Clinical Excellence.

http://guidance.nice.org.uk/CG92 Reducing the Risk of Venous Thromboembolism (Deep Vein Thrombosis and Pulmonary Embolism) in Patients Admitted to Hospital. (2010). National Institute of Health and Clinical Excellence.

http://guidance.nice.org.uk/CG48/Guidance/pdf/English MI: secondary prevention. (2007). National Institute of Health and Clinical Excellence.

www.rcgp.org.uk/PDF/ISH4[1].pdf Royal College of General Practitioners advice on safe warfarin therapy.

13. Blood Transfusion and Stem Cell Transplantation

http://nobelprize.org/educational_games/medicine/landsteiner/ An interactive blood-typing game.

www.learnbloodtransfusion.org.uk Better Blood Transfusion Continuing Education (NHS).

www.transfusionguidelines.org UK Blood Transfusion and Tissue Transplantation Services.

www.blood.co.uk NHS Blood and Transplant.

14. Things You Have to Know Before You Graduate

http://www.gmc-uk.org/education/undergraduate/tomorrows_doctors_2009.asp General Medical Council.

16

Preparing for Examinations and Self-Assessment

> ### Preparing for Exams
>
> ### Self-Assessment
>
> ☞ Basic multiple choice questions (MCQs)
> ☞ More advanced, single best answer multiple choice questions (SBA MCQs)
> ☞ Extended matching questions (EMQs)
> ☞ Answers to questions

Preparing for Exams

Remember that what you are really preparing for is a life-time commitment as a medical practitioner. You may see examinations as a barrier on the way but if they are well-designed examinations they will be testing core knowledge and skills that you need. Only some of these skills can be tested in a paper-based examination and that is all that can be dealt with here.

Work out ways that you find useful to tabulate and store basic knowledge for quick reference and revision. This is likely to be in electronic format but some people find light-weight cards are useful. Base your learning on actual patients. This makes knowledge more meaningful and therefore easier to remember. When you see a patient, make yourself familiar with the history and results of physical examination. Work out the differential diagnosis and the relevant tests and, when the tests results are available, make sure you can interpret them. Do some extra reading around the subject and see how theoretical knowledge can be applied to a clinical situation.

Ward rounds, outpatient clinics and clerking patients are all important. In the later years of your course make sure that you find out how to manage anticoagulant therapy and blood transfusions. Shadow the junior medical staff.

Self-Evaluation Questions

By the end of your haematology course you should know the approximate normal range in men and women for the haemoglobin concentration (Hb), mean cell volume (MCV), white cell count (WBC) and platelet count. If you need to refer to normal ranges for the full blood count and differential count to answer these questions see Tables 2.1 and 2.2, page 21 and 26.

Other useful ranges are shown in Table 16.1. NR = normal range. The most straightforward self-evaluation questions in this chapter are the basic multiple choice questions. The most difficult questions, requiring some clinical knowledge, are the extended matching questions; by the end of your medical course you should know the answer to almost all of these.

Basic Multiple Choice Questions

The number of true answers may be between 1 and 5.

Question 1

A high haemoglobin concentration could be the result of:

1. Renal carcinoma
2. Renal failure
3. Chronic obstructive pulmonary disease
4. Polycythaemia vera
5. Full and partial thickness burns over half the body

Table 16.1.   Normal ranges in adults.

Test	95% range
Vitamin B_{12}	180–640 ng/l
Serum folate	3–20 μg/l
Red cell folate	160–640 μg/l
Serum ferritin	15–300 μg/l
Serum iron	10–30 μmol/l
Serum transferrin	1.7–3.4 μ/l
Erythrocyte sedimentation rate	<10 mm in 1 hour (men),
	<15 mm in 1 hour (women)
Reticulocyte count	50–100 $\times$ 109/l
Haemoglobin A_2	2.0–3.5%
Prothrombin time	12–14 seconds
International normalised ratio	0.8–1.2
Activated partial thromboplastin time	30–40 seconds
Thrombin time	15–20 seconds
Fibrinogen assay	1.8–3.6 g/l
D-dimer	<200 mg/l
Serum bilirubin	<17 μmol/l
Alanine transaminase (ALT)	5–42 iu/l
Alkaline phosphatase	100–300 iu/l
Creatinine	60–125 μmol/l
Lactate dehydrogenase	200–450 iu/l
Calcium	2.15–2.55 mmol/l

Question 2

A 53-year-old woman is found to have a haemoglobin concentration of 10.1 g/dl and an MCV of 107 fl. This could be the result of:

1. Early iron deficiency
2. Excess alcohol intake
3. Myelodysplastic syndrome
4. Vitamin B_{12} deficiency
5. Hyperthyroidism

Question 3

An increased neutrophil count with toxic granulation is a likely result of:

1. Pneumococcal pneumonia
2. Gangrene of the foot
3. Infectious mononucleosis
4. Ethnic variation
5. Post-partum period

Question 4

A blood film might be expected to show spherocytes in:

1. Hereditary elliptocytosis
2. Autoimmune haemolytic anaemia
3. Delayed haemolytic transfusion reaction
4. Pregnancy
5. Iron deficiency anaemia

Question 5

A patient of blood group A Rh D-positive could safely receive a transfusion of red cells resuspended in SAGM from a donor who was:

1. Group AB Rh D-positive
2. Group A Rh D-negative
3. Group O Rh D-positive (high titre antibodies excluded)
4. Group B Rh D-positive
5. None of the above

Question 6

A 5-year-old boy presents with a haemarthrosis of the left knee. Coagulation studies show PT 14 s, aPTT 55 s, TT 18 s (control 19). Possible explanations of the coagulation defect include:

1. A defect in the intrinsic system
2. A defect in the extrinsic system

3. A defect in the common pathway
4. Thrombocytopenia
5. Hypofibrinogenaemia

(If necessary, refer to Fig. 11.1 to work out your answer)

Question 7

An 18-year-old man presents with a gastrointestinal haemorrhage. Coagulation studies show PT 13 s, aPTT 48 s, TT 18 s (control 20), fibrinogen concentration 3.7 g/l, D-dimer 158 mg/l (NR < 200). Likely explanations include:

1. Haemophilia A
2. Von Willebrand disease
3. Liver failure
4. Anticoagulant overdose
5. Disseminated intravascular coagulation

Question 8

Patients with long-standing difficult-to-control rheumatoid arthritis have an increased incidence of anaemia due to:

1. Iron deficiency
2. Felty's syndrome
3. Folic acid deficiency
4. Vitamin B_{12} deficiency
5. Anaemia of chronic disease

Question 9

A pregnant woman is blood group A Rh D-positive and her partner is group O Rh D-positive. The baby could be:

1. Group O Rh D-positive
2. Group O Rh-D negative

3. Group A Rh D-positive
4. Group A Rh-D negative
5. Group AB Rh-D negative

Question 10

A male surgical patient is blood group B Rh-D negative; he has never been transfused. The antibodies expected in his plasma are:

1. Anti-A
2. Anti-B
3. Anti-O
4. Anti D
5. Anti-d

Question 11

A high reticulocyte count could be due to:

1. Aplastic anaemia
2. Recent blood loss
3. Haemolysis
4. Chronic myeloid leukaemia
5. Untreated iron deficiency anaemia

Question 12

An 18-year-old student is febrile and his blood film shows numerous atypical lymphocytes. This could be due to:

1. Toxoplasmosis
2. An allergic reaction to a drug
3. Primary human immunodeficiency virus (HIV) infection
4. Primary cytomegalovirus (CMV) infection
5. Primary Epstein–Barr virus (EBV) infection

Single Best Answer Multiple Choice Questions

Question 13

A 66-year-old man had a blood count done while being monitored for hypercholesterolaemia and was found to have a lymphocyte count of $15.4 \times 10^9/l$ with the blood count being otherwise normal. The most likely diagnosis is:

1. Infectious mononucleosis
2. Cytomegalovirus infection
3. Acute lymphoblastic leukaemia
4. Pertussis
5. Chronic lymphocytic leukaemia

Question 14

A 23-year-old woman presents with a nose bleed and is found to have petechiae. A blood count shows a platelet count of $7 \times 10^9/l$, white cell count of $5.2 \times 10^9/l$ and haemoglobin concentration of 12.0 g/dl. The blood film does not show any platelet clumps or any other abnormality. A coagulation screen is normal. The most likely diagnosis is:

1. Human immunodeficiency virus (HIV) infection
2. Acute lymphoblastic leukaemia
3. Aplastic anaemia
4. Autoimmune thrombocytopenic purpura
5. Acute promyelocytic leukaemia

Question 15

A 35-year-old Scottish woman has a history of Crohn's disease with recent worsening of her symptoms. Her laboratory tests show: WBC $11.3 \times 10^9/l$, neutrophil count $9.3 \times 10^9/l$, lymphocyte count $1 \times 10^9/l$, monocyte count $1 \times 10^9/l$, Hb 9.7 g/dl, MCV 76 fl, platelet count $480 \times 10^9/l$, erythrocyte sedimentation rate 44 mm in 1 hour, serum iron 8 μmol/l (normal range [NR] 10–30), serum transferrin 1.5 g/l (NR 1.7–3.4) and serum ferritin 520 μg/l (15–300). The most likely cause of the anaemia is:

1. Vitamin B$_{12}$ deficiency due to Crohn's disease of the terminal ileum
2. Anaemia of chronic disease
3. Iron deficiency
4. Recent gastrointestinal blood loss
5. Folic acid deficiency

Question 16

A Greek couple both have a family history of thalassaemia and are therefore having pre-conceptual testing. They are both found to be heterozygous for β thalassaemia. The likely outcome of pregnancy in this couple is:

1. No risk of thalassaemia major
2. 25% chance of thalassaemia major
3. 50% chance of thalassaemia major
4. 75% chance of thalassaemia major
5. Thalassaemia major almost certain

Question 17

A 25-year-old Nigerian man requires emergency surgery following a road traffic accident causing multiple fractures. A blood count and sickle solubility test are performed. His Hb is 12.0 g/dl, a sickle solubility test is positive and a blood film shows some target cells. Which statement is true?

1. He has sickle cell heterozygosity, which is of no significance
2. He has sickle cell anaemia and surgery should not be undertaken
3. He has sickle cell heterozygosity and care must be taken to avoid hypoxia, dehydration and acidosis
4. No diagnosis can be made without further tests so surgery should be delayed

5. He has sickle cell anaemia and surgery should not be undertaken without an exchange transfusion

Question 18

A 56-year-old man presents with numbness in his feet and is found to have reduced vibration sense and joint position sense. Plantar responses are upgoing. A blood count shows an Hb of 11.8 g/dl and an MCV of 103 fl. The most likely explanation is:

1. Diabetic neuropathy
2. Folic acid deficiency
3. Multiple sclerosis
4. Spinal cord compression
5. Pernicious anaemia

Question 19

The normal intravascular life span of a neutrophil is about:

1. One hour
2. Seven hours
3. Twenty-four hours
4. Ten days
5. 120 days

Question 20

A 35-year-old Indian vegetarian woman with three young children complains of fatigue and is found to have an Hb of 8 g/dl. Her blood film shows hypochromia, microcytosis and pencil cells (elliptocytes). The most likely diagnosis is:

1. Hereditary elliptocytosis
2. Vitamin B_{12} deficiency
3. Iron deficiency anaemia
4. Lead poisoning
5. Folic acid deficiency

Question 21

An Eritrean refugee is investigated for iron deficiency anaemia and is found to have hookworm. His blood film is most likely to show:

1. Neutrophilia
2. Eosinophilia
3. Basophilia
4. Lymphocytosis
5. Monocytosis

Question 22

A 50-year-old man suffers a crushing central chest pain radiating to his left shoulder. The next day he is found to have a leucocytosis (WBC $13 \times 10^9/l$) and neutrophilia (neutrophil count $8.5 \times 10^9/l$). The Hb and platelet count are normal. The most likely explanation of the abnormality in the blood count is:

1. Chronic myelogenous leukaemia
2. Myocardial infarction
3. Pneumococcal pneumonia
4. Splenic infarction
5. Aortic dissection

Question 23

The Accident and Emergency Department requires fresh-frozen plasma for a 66-year-old man of unknown blood group who appears to have very impaired liver function and is bleeding from oesophageal varices. Which group plasma would be chosen?

1. O
2. A
3. B
4. AB
5. None of the above

Question 24

A 46-year-old woman presents with weight loss and abdominal enlargement. She has also noticed that she is sweating more than normal and her temperature is 38°C. She is found to have enlargement of the liver 2 cm below the right costal margin and of the spleen 6 cm below the left costal margin. Lymph nodes are not enlarged. FBC shows: WBC $98 \times 10^9/l$, Hb 8.3 g/dl and platelet count $504 \times 10^9/l$. A blood film shows increased numbers of neutrophils, eosinophils and basophils. In addition white cell precursors are increased although blast cells are infrequent. The optimal treatment for this patient is likely to be:

1. Allogeneic stem cell transplantation
2. Combination chemotherapy
3. Imatinib
4. Blood transfusion as required to relieve symptoms
5. Rifampicin and isoniazid

Extended Matching Questions

Question 25

Theme

Abnormalities of white cells.

Option list

A. Acute lymphoblastic leukaemia
B. Acute myeloid leukaemia
C. Acute promyelocytic leukaemia
D. Chronic lymphocytic leukaemia
E. Chronic myelogenous leukaemia (Philadelphia-positive)
F. Follicular lymphoma
H. Hodgkin lymphoma
I. Reactive lymphocytosis
J. Reactive neutrophilia

For each clinical history below, choose the most appropriate and specific diagnosis from the list above. Each option may be used once, more than once or not at all.

1. A 54-year-old man presents with weight loss and increased sweating. His spleen is felt 8 cm below his left costal margin. His FBC shows: WBC 111.2×10^9/l, Hb 9.5 g/dl, platelet count 540×10^9/l. A differential count shows a marked increase in neutrophils and neutrophil precursors but blast cells are infrequent. Eosinophils and basophils are also increased.

2. A 4-year-old boy is noted by his mother to be pale and listless. His general practitioner finds him to have cervical and inguinal lymphadenopathy and several bruises on his legs. FBC shows: WBC 49.5×10^9/l with 85% blast cells, Hb 8.5 g/dl, platelet count 48×10^9/l. The blast cells have no granules.

3. A 75-year-old man presents with herpes zoster. FBC shows: WBC 18×10^9/l, Hb 15.5 g/dl, platelet count 200×10^9/l, lymphocyte count 12.3×10^9/l. The blood film shows mature small lymphocytes.

4. A 50-year-old woman presents with pallor and bruising. Her spleen is felt 2 cm below her left costal margin and some petechiae are noted. She is febrile and has moist sounds at both lung bases. FBC shows: WBC 16.8×10^9/l, Hb 8.5 g/dl, platelet count 80×10^9/l. The blood film shows that about 50% of leucocytes are blast cells, some of which contain Auer rods.

5. A 48-year-old woman has previously been treated for carcinoma of the breast by removal of the breast lump, radiotherapy and chemotherapy. She presents 6 years later with epistaxis, extensive bruising and haemorrhage into soft tissues of her arms. Her FBC shows: WBC 6.3×10^9/l with neutrophilia, Hb 11.6 g/dl, platelet count 45×10^9/l. Her blood film shows small numbers of immature cells that are packed with brightly staining granules. A coagulation screen shows prolonged prothrombin time, activated partial thromboplastin time and thrombin time. Fibrinogen concentration is reduced and fibrin degradation products are increased.

Question 26

Theme

Renal disease.

Option list

A. Carcinoma of the kidney
B. Glomerulonephritis
C. Haemolytic uraemic syndrome
D. Hyperparathyroidism
E. Loss of renal concentrating ability
F. Monoclonal gammopathy of undetermined significance
G. Multiple myeloma
H. Renal failure due to recurrent infarction
I. Thrombotic thrombocytopenic purpura
J. Wegener's granulomatosus

For each clinical history below, choose the most appropriate diagnosis from the list above. Each option may be used once, more than once or not at all.

1. A 4-year-old girl presents with jaundice and pallor that followed an episode of diarrhoea. Her FBC shows: WBC 11.2×10^9/l, Hb 8.4 g/dl, platelet count 352×10^9/l. Her blood film shows numerous red cell fragments and polychromasia. Her creatinine and potassium are elevated.

2. A 44-year-old woman presents with fever, purpura and mental confusion. There is no lymphadenopathy or hepatosplenomegaly. FBC shows: WBC 13.8×10^9/l, Hb 8.7 g/dl, platelet count 52×10^9/l. The blood film shows numerous schistocytes. Creatinine is elevated.

3. A 45-year-old man has a life-time history of sickle cell anaemia. FBC shows: WBC 6.8×10^9/l, Hb 5.0 g/dl, platelet count 243×10^9/l. The blood film shows sickle cells, target cells and Howell–Jolly bodies. Creatinine is elevated and reticulocyte count is not increased.

4. A 56-year-old man presents with fatigue and haematuria. A mass in found in the right loin. FBC shows: WBC 12.8×10^9/l, Hb 18.5 g/dl,

platelet count 400×10^9/l. The blood film is reported as showing a 'packed film.'

5. A 63-year-old man presents with back ache, which has been troubling him for several months. No specific abnormality is found on physical examination. His FBC shows: WBC 6.7×10^9/l, Hb 9.6 g/dl, platelet count 145×10^9/l. His blood film shows rouleaux and increased background staining and erythrocyte sedimentation rate is 78 mm in one hour. He has an elevated calcium and creatinine.

Question 27

Theme

Anticoagulant therapy.

Option list

A. INR is appropriate for this patient
B. INR is too high, give fresh-frozen plasma
C. INR is too high, give fresh-frozen plasma and vitamin K
D. INR is too high, give oral vitamin K
E. INR is too high, give protamine sulphate
F. INR is too high, reduce dose of warfarin
G. INR is too low, give heparin
H. INR is too low, increase warfarin dose

For each warfarinised patient choose the most appropriate action from the option list above in the light of the International normalised ratio (INR) result.

1. A patient with a prosthetic mitral valve has an INR of 3.0
2. A patient who is on warfarin following a post-operative deep vein thrombosis 3 months earlier suffers a gastrointestinal haemorrhage and is found to have an INR of 4.5
3. A patient with a prosthetic aortic valve has an INR of 1.8
4. A patient with atrial fibrillation has an INR of 4.0
5. A patient with a prosthetic mitral valve has an INR of 4.0

Question 28

Theme

Sickle cell disease.

Option list

A. Acute chest crisis
B. Dactylitis
C. Osteomyelitis
D. Painful crisis
E. Parvovirus-induced red cell aplasia
F. Pneumococcal pneumonia
G. Septic arthritis
H. Splenic infarction
I. Splenic sequestration
J. Splenic vein thrombosis

For each patient with sickle cell anaemia select from the option list above the most likely explanation of the clinical picture.

1. A 2-year-old child presents with pallor and marked lethargy, an Hb of 4 g/dl and enlargement of the spleen to below the umbilicus.
2. A 7-year-old and her 5-year old sister present with pallor and lassitude. Both are found to have had a fall of Hb and their reticulocyte counts are considerably below the normal range.
3. A 2-year-old presents with acute swelling of one hand and one foot. She is crying with pain.
4. A 4-year-old child has left upper quadrant and left shoulder tip pain. His spleen is felt on inspiration and is tender.
5. A 10-year-old child presents with rib and abdominal pain with no specific localising signs.

Question 29

Theme

Splenomegaly.

Option list

A. Acquired immune deficiency syndrome
B. Acute lymphoblastic leukaemia
C. Amyloidosis of the spleen
D. Biliary cirrhosis
E. Chronic lymphocytic leukaemia
F. Haemochromatosis
G. Hodgkin lymphoma
H. Metastatic carcinoma
I. Portal cirrhosis
J. Primary myelofibrosis

For each clinical history select the most likely diagnosis form the option list above.

1. A 32-year-old engineer presents with fever, night sweats and itch. He is found to have generalised lymphadenopathy (nodes 1.5–2 cm) and his spleen is felt 3 cm below the left costal margin. FBC and bio-chemical tests show a normocytic normochromic anaemia with the biochemical features of anaemia of chronic disease. He has eosinophilia and his erythrocyte sedimentation rate is increased.

2. A 65-year-old accountant presents to his general practitioner because of impotence. He does not smoke and rarely takes any alcohol. He is noted to be heavily pigmented, his liver is abnormally firm and his spleen is just felt below the left costal margin. There is no lymph node enlargement. An FBC shows anaemia and thrombocytopenia. His blood film shows no specific abnormalities.

3. A 67-year-old retired school teacher presents with abdominal enlarge-ment and bruising. He is found to be pale with enlargement of the spleen 8 cm below the left costal margin. An FBC shows: WBC $3.8 \times 10^9/l$, Hb 9.0 g/dl, platelet count $82 \times 10^9/l$. The blood film is leucoerythroblastic and shows anisocytosis and poikilocytosis includ-ing teardrop poikilocytes.

4. A 69-year-old retired man who is being followed up for hypertension is found to have generalised lymphadenopathy with lymph nodes up to 1.5 cm in diameter. His spleen is felt 2 cm below the left costal

margin. An FBC shows: WBC $54 \times 10^9/l$, lymphocyte count $48 \times 10^9/l$, Hb 11 g/dl and platelet count $110 \times 10^9/l$. The lymphocytes are small and mature and smear cells are present.

5. A 54-year-old ex-stockbroker presents with abdominal enlargement. He smokes 15 cigarettes per day and reports taking 5–6 units of alcohol per day. He is found to have ascites, splenomegaly, a firm irregular liver edge, gynaecomastia and testicular atrophy. There are no palpable lymph nodes. FBC shows mild pancytopenia and macrocytosis; blood film shows no abnormal cells.

Question 30

Theme

Anaemia.

Options

A. Anaemia of chronic disease
B. Autoimmune haemolytic anaemia
C. Glucose-6-phosphate dehydrogenase deficiency
D. Hereditary spherocytosis
E. Iron deficiency anaemia
F. Megaloblastic anaemia
G. Myelodysplastic syndrome
H. Sickle cell anaemia
I. Sickle cell heterozygosity
J. Thalassaemia intermedia

1. A 50-year-old Northern European Caucasian man notices altered bowel function and is found to have an Hb of 8.8 g/dl and an MCV of 70 fl. His diet is normal.
2. A 16-year-old African boy presents with haematuria. His WBC is $4.5 \times 10^9/l$, Hb 12.5 g/dl and platelet count $423 \times 10^9/l$. His blood film shows target cells. A sickle solubility test is positive.
3. A 34-year-old Northern European woman with a history of systemic lupus erythematosus presents with jaundice and fatigue.

She is found to have an increase of unconjugated bilirubin and lactate dehydrogenase, an Hb of 9.5 g/dl, spherocytes and an increased reticulocyte count. Her direct antiglobulin test is positive.

4. A 23-year-old Italian man is given antibiotics for a urinary tract infection and a few days later presents with the acute onset of jaundice, pallor, fatigue and breathlessness. He is found to have an Hb of 6.2 g/dl and an increased reticulocyte count and a blood film showing numerous irregularly contracted cells.

5. A 53-year-old French woman present with fatigue and is found to have an Hb of 8.8 g/dl and an MCV of 110 fl. Neutrophils show reduced segmentation (pseudo-Pelger-Huët anomaly) and are hypogranular. Platelet count is 60×10^9/l. Vitamin B_{12} and folic acid assays are normal.

Answers to Questions

Basic Multiple Choice Questions

Question 1

1, 3, 4 and 5 are true. Renal failure causes a low haemoglobin concentration.

Question 2

2, 3 and 4 are correct. Iron deficiency causes microcytosis. It is hypothyroidism that can cause a macrocytic anaemia, not hyperthyroidism.

Question 3

1, 2 and 5 are correct. Infectious mononucleosis causes an increase of atypical lymphocytes and neutropenia rather than neutrophilia is an ethnic variation.

Question 4

2 and 3 are correct. The spherocytosis is because sections of the antibody-coated red cell membrane have been removed by splenic macrophages.

Question 5

2 and 3 are correct but remember that it would generally be preferable to keep A D-negative red cells for D-negative recipients.

Question 6

1 is correct. This can only be a defect in the intrinsic system since the PT is normal. The likely diagnoses are haemophilia (factor VIII deficiency) and factor IX deficiency.

Question 7

The defect can be localised to the intrinsic pathway. Either 1 (haemophilia A) or 2 (von Willebrand disease) is likely. In von Willebrand disease the prolonged APTT is because of the associated reduction in factor VIII clotting activity.

Question 8

1, 2 and 5 are true. The likelihood of iron deficiency is increased because the patient may have been taking aspirin, non-steroidal anti-inflammatory drugs or corticosteroids, any of which could cause chronic gastrointestinal blood loss. Felty's syndrome is a complication of rheumatoid arthritis in which both hypersplenism and autoantibodies contribute to anaemia and cytopenia (particularly neutropenia).

Question 9

1, 2, 3 and 4 are true. (Remember that group A may be genetically OA and group D may be genetically Dd.)

Question 10

1 is true. Only anti-A is expected. Anti-O and anti-d do not exist and anti-D is not expected in a man who has never been transfused.

Question 11

2 and 3 are true. In the other conditions the bone marrow is unable to make an appropriate response to anaemia.

Question 12

All answers are true.

Single Best Answer Multiple Choice Questions

Question 13

The most likely diagnosis is chronic lymphocytic leukaemia (5). None of the other conditions is likely to cause lymphocytosis in an asymptomatic middle-aged man.

Question 14

The most likely diagnosis is autoimmune thrombocytopenic purpura (ITP; 4) as the other diagnoses are less likely to cause isolated very severe thrombocytopenia. The only other diagnosis that should be seriously considered is acute promyelocytic leukaemia, but the normal haemoglobin concentration and the normal coagulation screen make this less likely than ITP.

Question 15

The anaemia is most likely anaemia of chronic disease (2) as a result of her inflammatory bowel disease. This is suggested by the low iron and transferrin and the raised ferritin.

Question 16

There is a 25% chance of β thalassaemia major (2) with each conception in this couple.

Question 17

The mild anaemia is consistent with blood loss. The near normal Hb and the fact that the blood film shows only target cells makes sickle cell anaemia very unlikely. The most likely diagnosis is sickle cell trait (3), which requires particular care with anaesthesia.

Question 18

The most likely diagnosis is pernicious anaemia (5). Patients who present with neurological features may have only mild haematological abnormalities.

Question 19

The normal intravascular life span of a neutrophil is about 7 hours (2). 10 days is the life span of a platelet and 120 days the life span of a red cell.

Question 20

Vegetarians, particularly women who have had a number of pregnancies, are much more likely to have iron deficiency (3) than vitamin B_{12} deficiency and neither B_{12} deficiency nor folic acid deficiency would explain the blood film. Some elliptocytes can be seen in iron deficiency and hereditary elliptocytosis would not explain the hypochromia and microcytosis. Lead poisoning can cause a microcytic anaemia but is quite uncommon.

Question 21

His blood film is most likely to show eosinophilia (2).

Question 22

The most likely explanation is myocardial infarction (2) causing reactive neutrophilia.

Question 23

Group AB plasma (4) would be selected for a patient of unknown group who required urgent correction of a coagulation defect.

Question 24

This is a complex question since it requires the right diagnosis to be made so that the optimal treatment can be selected. The patient is likely to have chronic myelogenous leukaemia and the optimal treatment is therefore imatinib (3).

Extended Matching Questions

Question 25

1E, 2A, 3D, 4B, 5C (Note that 5B is also correct but you are asked for the most appropriate specific diagnosis.)

Question 26

1C, 2I, 3H, 4A, 5G.

Question 27

1A, 2C, 3H, 4F, 5A.

Question 28

1I, 2E, 3B, 4H, 5D.

Question 29

1G, 2F, 3J, 4E, 5I.

Question 30

1E, 2I, 3B, 4C, 5G.

17

Answers to Test Cases

Test Case 3.1

There is nothing to suggest any chronic infection of active inflammation and the borderline elevation of the erythrocyte sedimentation rate (ESR) and C-reactive protein (CRP) is against this possibility. This is therefore likely to be iron deficiency anaemia. The next test to be done is serum ferritin, which was done and confirmed iron deficiency. The patient can be treated with oral ferrous sulphate but his management must also include finding out the cause of the iron deficiency. He has been taking aspirin regularly so chronic blood loss from the stomach is possible. However, in a man of this age the possibility of colonic carcinoma must not be neglected. He requires a colonoscopy. This was performed and showed a carcinoma of the ascending colon. This may be the reason for the slight elevation of the CRP (it has been found to be increased, on average, in patients with colonic cancer).

Test Case 4.1

The most likely diagnosis is pernicious anaemia since the neurological symptoms are consistent with vitamin B_{12} deficiency and there is also macrocytosis. Pernicious anaemia is the most likely cause of an overt vitamin B_{12} deficiency in a middle-aged or elderly Caucasian woman with a normal diet. Although excess alcohol intake can cause peripheral neuropathy, 1–2 units a day is not sufficient to do this. Some patients under-report their alcohol intake but the normal liver function tests in this patient make alcohol excess unlikely. Hypothyroidism has not been excluded as a cause of the macrocytosis but would not explain all the neurological abnormalities.

Serum vitamin B_{12} and red cell folate should be assayed and intrinsic factor antibodies should be sought. Serum B_{12} is very likely to be low and red cell folate may also be reduced. It is quite likely that intrinsic factor antibodies will be detected. The patient is likely to be treated with parenteral hydroxocobalamin, starting with 1,000 μg daily in view of the neurological deficit. Her maintenance dose will be 1,000 μg each 3 months.

Test Case 5.1

Gallstones are surprising at this age and are the result of increased bilirubin production caused by a chronic haemolytic anaemia. The most likely diagnosis is hereditary spherocytosis. Spherocytes could also be due to autoimmune haemolytic anaemia but this is unlikely for two reasons. First, it is unlikely that the patient has had an undiagnosed autoimmune haemolytic anaemia for such a long time that gallstones have developed. Second, the direct antiglobulin test is negative, so there is no evidence of immunoglobulin or complement on the red cell membrane.

Test Case 5.2

The very low reticulocyte count and the lack of polychromasia is not something that we would normally expect in sickle cell anaemia, since the marrow responds to the shortened red cell life span by an increased output of erythrocytes. This suggests failure of erythropoiesis. Megaloblastic anaemia is unlikely because folic acid is being taken regularly and the white cell and platelet counts are normal. This is most likely pure red cell aplasia as a result of parvovirus B19 infection. The anaemia is severe so blood transfusion is needed after first taking a blood sample to test for antibodies to parvovirus.

Test Case 6.1

The first thing to consider is whether the patient has pancytopenia as a result of bone marrow metastases. However, the blood film is not leuco-erythroblastic and there are no biochemical abnormalities to suggest widespread metastases. What the blood film does show is dysplastic neutrophils, red cells features that suggest sideroblastic erythropoiesis and occasional blast cells. The most likely diagnosis is myelodysplastic syndrome resulting from previous chemotherapy. The previous medical history is certainly relevant. The patient would have a bone marrow aspirate and cytogenetic analysis performed and the nature of the condition and the prognosis would be discussed with her. As her anaemia is symptomatic, a trial of erythropoietin could be considered as a first step.

Test Case 7.1

The red cell indices suggest that the patient has iron deficiency anaemia. The eosinophil count is increased. Hookworm infection would provide an explanation of both the iron deficiency and the eosinophilia. Being an asylum-seeker from an impoverished country there might also be dietary deficiency. In a Somalian, schistosomiasis could also be considered as a cause of eosinophilia. If you looked up a normal range for the neutrophil count you might consider that this is a low neutrophil count. However, in a Somalian it could be normal, i.e. an ethnic neutropenia.

Test Case 7.2

The patient has carbimazole-induced agranulocytosis. The carbimazole should be stopped immediately, blood and throat swabs should be taken for culture, and antibiotics should be prescribed. Agranulocytosis is a serious illness and if the patient is febrile, hospitalisation is indicated. Administration of granulocyte colony-stimulating factor could be considered as it may shorten the period of agranulocytosis.

Test Case 8.1

The findings are those of chronic lymphocytic leukaemia (CLL). There is a clone of kappa-positive B cells present, expressing surface membrane immunoglobulin weakly. There are a small number of lambda-positive normal B cells and 10% of cells are T cells. CD5 is expressed on the great majority of cells so clearly is being expressed on the ~85% of clonal B cells as well as the T cells. The neoplastic cells therefore expressed weak immunoglobulin, CD5 and CD23 but not FMC7 or CD79b. The patient has early disease so he does not need any chemotherapy. However, he could be vaccinated against pneumococcus and start annual influenza vaccination.

Test Case 8.2

The findings suggest acute lymphoblastic leukaemia (ALL). On the data given it is not possible to totally exclude acute myeloid leukaemia with very primitive myeloblasts that do not express peroxidase (FAB M0 AML). However, the fact that there is mediastinal enlargement is very suggestive of T-lineage ALL, so the immunophenotyping is likely to confirm T-ALL and exclude M0 AML. Other tests needed are biochemical screening (tests of renal and liver function, uric acid, calcium, phosphate), blood group and antibody screen, and bone marrow aspiration for cytogenetic analysis.

Test Case 9.1

The combination of a high haemoglobin concentration (Hb) and a *JAK2* V617F mutation is sufficient to make the diagnosis of polycythaemia vera. This can be suspected from the blood count and film alone because of the combination of polycythaemia, neutrophilia, basophilia and thrombocytosis. There are no other essential tests. The patient should be managed by lowering the Hb. Because of the recent cerebrovascular accident it would be prudent to accompany the initial venesections with infusion of normal saline solution to protect the patient from changing blood volume and possible hypotension. Once the Hb has been lowered to a safe level, hydroxycarbamide would be an ideal form of ongoing management as that will also control the thrombocytosis. Aspirin 75 mg daily should be prescribed.

Test Case 10.1

The plasma cell percentage in the bone marrow is not very high (remember that the distribution of myeloma cell in the marrow may be patchy) but the level of the paraprotein, the lytic lesion in the clavicle and the presence of anaemia indicate that this is myeloma. It is not extramedullary myeloma since there is both a clavicular lesion and bone marrow disease detected on marrow aspiration. The clavicular lesion and the anaemia also mean that it is symptomatic rather than asymptomatic myeloma.

Test Case 11.1

Obstruction of the common bile duct has occurred as a result of growth of the pancreatic cancer, leading to a deficiency of fat-soluble vitamins, including vitamin K, and the vitamin K-dependent factors, II, VII, IX and X. The fibrinogen is increased as a non-specific response to the tumour.

Test Case 11.2

There is a history of mucosal bleeding, an apparent autosomal dominant inheritance and a deficiency of factor VIII and von Willebrand factor in a woman. This points to a diagnosis of von Willebrand disease. The bleeding time would be likely to be prolonged as von Willebrand factor is one of the mechanisms binding platelets to exposed subendothelial collagen. Factor VIII is low because von Willebrand factor stabilises factor VIII and increases its half-life in the plasma.

Test Case 12.1

The combination of a spontaneous venous thrombosis and prolonged APTT suggest a lupus anticoagulant. There is a suspicion that the patient actually has systemic lupus erythematosus in view of the history of arthritis and the neutropenia and thrombocytopenia. Laboratory tests are needed to confirm the presence of a lupus anticoagulant. She also requires testing for antinuclear activity and anti-dsDNA antibodies. Renal function should be checked and the urine should be tested for albumin. The patient requires anticoagulation. This could be initially with low molecular weight heparin overlapping with warfarin. The warfarin should continue long term. She should be closely monitored for symptoms and signs of bleeding in view of the associated moderate thrombocytopenia. Consideration could be given to the use of low molecular weight heparin rather than warfarin if there were any particular risk factors for haemorrhage associated with warfarin.

Abbreviation: dsDNA, double-stranded deoxynucleic acid.

Test Case 13.1

An ABO-incompatible transfusion should be suspected. Stop the transfusion immediately but keep the drip open and maintain the blood pressure and the urine output by infusion of normal saline. Check the patient's identity and check the details on the bag of blood in comparison with the wrist band and the blood request form. If you find that the wrong bag of blood was being transfused, check urgently that the bag intended for this patient is not being given to another patient in the Day Case Ward. Inform the transfusion laboratory and return the bag of blood immediately to the transfusion laboratory together with a further blood sample from the patient, which will be used to confirm the group, repeat the antibody screen and perform a direct antiglobulin test. At the same time, take a sample to check liver and renal function, electrolytes and coagulation status. Ask the nursing staff to test the next urine sample that the patient passes for blood. Phone a member of the hospital transfusion team or a consultant haematologist for advice and help.

Index